Family Dinner Cookbook

A Variety of 180+ Quick & Easy Dinner Recipes That Are So Delicious the Whole Family Will Love Them!

by Olivia Rogers

Copyright © 2017 By Olivia Rogers
All rights reserved. No part of this book may be reproduced in any form without permission in writing from the author. No part of this publication may be reproduced or transmitted in any form or by any means, mechanic, electronic, photocopying, recording, by any storage or retrieval system, or transmitted by email without the permission in writing from the author and publisher.
For information regarding permissions write to author at
Olivia@TheMenuAtHome.com
Reviewers may quote brief passages in review.

Please note that credit for the images used in this book go to the respective owners. You can view this at: TheMenuAtHome.com/image-list

Olivia Rogers
TheMenuAtHome.com

Table of Contents

Introduction *11*
Who is this book for? *11*
What will this book teach you? *11*
1. Low Carb Pot Roast Swaddled in Bacon *12*
2. Cheesy Hot Tuna Melt Platter *13*
3. Seared Broccoli with a Lemon Twist *13*
4. British Pork Cutlet Dressed in Cumberland Sauce *14*
5. Savory Broccoli, Ginger and Sesame Stir Fry *15*
6. Monumental Meatloaf *17*
7. Aunt Sally's Savory Sausage Scramble *18*
8. Mamma's Mushroom and Green Bean Mishmash *19*
9. Mushroom Mayhem *20*
10. Spooky Pumpkin Seeds with Baked Chicken *21*
11. Tummy Tempting Tomato Salsa with Roast Beef *22*
12. Happy Humming Hummus with Pita Bread *22*
13. Texan Scramble *23*
14. Chicken Salad *24*
15. Shrimp & Avocado Salad *25*
16. Coconut Pancakes *26*
17. Shrimp, Leek, and Spinach Pasta *27*
18. Spicy Salmon and Rice *28*
19. Chicken, Zucchini with Prosciutto *28*
20. Pecorino Chicken *29*
21. The Classic Chicken Curry *30*
22. The Classic Grilled Cheese Sandwich *31*

23. Slow Cooker Roast Chicken _____ 32
24. Barbequed Beef Sandwiches _____ 32
25. Baked Spaghetti _____ 33
26. Pork Chops with Apples _____ 34
27. Red Potato Salad _____ 35
28. Chili Coke Roast _____ 36
29. Chicken Stroganoff _____ 37
30. Lamb Chops and Peppercorns _____ 38
31. Roasted Chicken with Honey Glazed Sweet Potatoes _____ 39
32. Mushroom Potato Gratin _____ 40
33. Meatball Mash _____ 41
34. Smoked Turkey with Almond Mole _____ 43
35. Stuffed Chicken Rolls _____ 44
36. Juicy Make Ahead Ribs _____ 45
37. Stuffed Lasagna Rolls _____ 46
38. Prosciutto Wrapped Chicken with Pesto Pasta _____ 47
39. Make Ahead Pierogies _____ 48
40. Almond Crusted Chicken Casserole _____ 49
41. Make Ahead Quiche _____ 51
42. Sausage Manicotti _____ 52
43. Onion Pepper Sausage Calzone _____ 53
44. Hearty Chicken & Noodle Soup _____ 54
45. Beef & Barley Soup _____ 55
46. Mushroom Soup with Herbed Cream _____ 56
47. Cozy Butternut Squash Soup _____ 57
48. Herbed Pork & Beans _____ 58
49. Green Chili _____ 59

50. Rich & Hearty Pork Stew _____ 60
51. Guinness Beef Stew _____ 62
52. Make Ahead Beef Rolls _____ 63
53. Black Bean & Sweet Potato Empanadas _____ 64
54. Make Ahead Samosas _____ 65
5. Sweet Potato Burritos _____ 66
56. Quick Wraps _____ 68
57. Cheesy Chive Loaf _____ 69
58. Buttermilk Whole Grain Pancakes _____ 70
59. Cherry Chocolate Cookies _____ 71
60. Lamb Tagine _____ 72
61. Crispy Bacon with Cauliflower Pasta _____ 73
62. Fishy Fish Pie _____ 74
63. Eggplant and Sausages _____ 75
64. Chili Pasta with Cauliflowers _____ 76
65. Different Mac n Cheese _____ 77
66. Easy Cheese Pizza _____ 78
67. Easy Tomato Soup _____ 79
68. Turkey Burgers _____ 80
69. Chicken Curry with Sweet Potatoes _____ 81
70. Ratatouille Salad _____ 82
71. Bean and Sausages in a Pot _____ 83
72. Chili Cheese Mac n Cheese _____ 84
73. Pita Pockets _____ 85
74. Pesto Sandwiches _____ 86
75. Baked Dish with Veggies _____ 87
76. Shrimp and Spinach Pasta _____ 88

77. Shrimp and Olive Salad	89
78. Asian Salmon with Bok Choy	90
79. Salmon and Fennel Salad	90
80. Chicken with Prosciutto	91
81. Turkey and Broccoli Pasta	92
82. Beef Chili	94
83. Kale and Tomato Spaghetti	95
84. Poached Fish	96
85. Green Grape Curry	97
86. Spanish Omelets	98
87. Baked Cod	99
88. Sausage Stir-Fry	100
89. Chicken Mince Cutlets	101
90. Chickpea Salad	102
91. Citrus Fish	103
92. Tomato Spiced Risotto	104
93. Pesto Pasta	105
94. Tenderloin with Salsa	106
95. Seriously Sloppy Joe's	107
96. Pasta with Chunky Meat Sauce	108
97. Lamb and Veg Stew	109
98. Mushroom Soup with Barley	110
99. Bean Soup with Sausages	111
100. Fish with Tomato Olive Salsa	112
101. Shrimp Noodle Soup	113
102. Pesto Soup with Chickpeas	114
103. Chorizo Pea Soup	115

104. Tomato Bruschetta's	115
105. Aubergine Sandwiches	116
106. Chicken Burritos	117
107. British Fish and Chips	118
108. BBQ Chicken Sandwich	119
109. Tuna and Caper Sandwich	120
110. Creamy Zucchini Pasta	121
111. Pork with Cabbage Noodles	122
112. Thai Soup	123
113. Cauliflower Soup	124
114. Apple Cheese Sandwiches	125
115. Sambal Chicken Sandwiches	126
116. Pesto Tuna Subway	126
117. Egg and Prosciutto Panini	127
118. Chicken Noodles	128
119. Peas Pasta	129
120. Simple Chocolate Cheesecake	130
121. Garden Pasta Salad	131
122. Texas Coleslaw	132
123. Potato Salad	133
124. Picnic Summer Slaw	134
125. Sweet Corn and Tomato Salad	134
126. Pork Tenderloin and Cucumber Salad	135
127. Great American Potato Salad	136
128. Olive Caprese Salad	137
129. Cheese Burger Bites	138
130. Spicy Peanuts	139

131. Grilled Vegetable Skewers with Pesto Vinaigrette _____ 139
132. Grilled Zucchini Rolls with Bacon and Cheese _____ 141
133. Seven Layer Dip _____ 141
134. Italian Skewers _____ 142
135. Cornmeal Tarts with Cheese _____ 143
136. Sesame Salmon Croquettes _____ 144
137. Deviled Eggs _____ 145
138. Rancho Baked Beans _____ 146
139. Mexican Corn Bread _____ 146
140. Baconista Brats _____ 147
141. Texas Cowboy Style Ribs _____ 148
142. Grilled Corn with Chili and Manchego Cheese _____ 150
143. Dressed Up Bacon Mac and Cheese _____ 150
144. Garlicky Summer Squash and Fresh Corn _____ 151
145. Daddy's Fried Corn and Onion _____ 152
146. Baked 3-Bean Casserole _____ 153
147. Grilled Mussels _____ 154
148. Gazpacho _____ 154
149. Tuna & Eggplant Salad in a Jar _____ 156
150. Peanut Butter & Berry Pie _____ 157
151. Plum Semifreddo _____ 158
152. Cherry Bourbon Ice Cream _____ 159
153. Open Faced Eggplant & Basil Sandwiches _____ 160
154. Corn Zucchini Feta Salad _____ 161
155. Buttery Salmon with Hazelnut Relish _____ 162
156. Steak Okra Tomato Kebabs _____ 163
157. Pork Chops Topped with Pickled Watermelon Salad _____ 165

158. Porterhouse Steak with Herbed Butter _____ 166
159. Grilled Panzanella _____ 167
160. Zucchini Patties _____ 168
161. Chicken Salad with Crème Fraiche and Rye _____ 169
162. Lobster Spaghetti _____ 170
163. Melon Soup _____ 171
164. Pan-Fried Shishito Peppers _____ 172
165. Sweet & Savory Summer Salad _____ 173
166. Summery Spinach _____ 174
167. Avocado Plum Salad _____ 175
168. Summer Picnic Rolls _____ 176
169. Sweet Corn Soup _____ 177
170. Summer Slaw _____ 179
171. Marinated Summer Veggies _____ 180
172. Pan-Fried Summer Squash _____ 181
173. Berry Pudding _____ 182
174. Corn & Cod Chowder _____ 183
175. Fruit Cobbler _____ 184
176. Summer Stir Fry _____ 185
177. Summery Linguine _____ 186
178. Summer Tarts _____ 187
179. Summer Garden Tortellini _____ 188
180. Summer Kebabs _____ 189
181. Squash Sloppy Joes _____ 190
182. Drunken Shaved Ice _____ 192
183. Mint Hot Fudge Sundaes _____ 192
184. Whiskey Wings _____ 194

185. Fruit Salad in Herbed Syrup	*195*
186. Blueberry Banana Bread	*196*
187. Frozen Peach Yogurt	*197*
Final Words	*198*
Disclaimer	*199*

Introduction

I have put together a total of quick and easy recipes to help you stage the dinner table for your family. Now, you don't have to waste your time thinking about the perfect recipe. You have it all in one place for you! Many of us want to eat better but we just don't have the time or energy to cook after work. It's easy to give in to the temptation of delivery or unhealthy TV dinners after a long day at the office.

When you cook everything ahead of time and then just store it in the freezer, you can eat healthy, satisfying meals every day of the week. Each of these delicious recipes you'll find in this book are perfect for preparing ahead of time and freezing until you are ready to eat. For each recipe, you will notice that one step is written in italics. This means that if you are planning to freeze the meal for later, this is the step after which you'll store it in the freezer. If there are additional steps after, do those right before you plan to eat the meal.

The recipes mentioned in this book are all healthy family meals, which don't take too much time to make, and are also attractive to the children within the family. Each recipe comes with additional tips or interesting facts about the dish itself, allowing you to take more interest in it overall. All the recipes mentioned in this book satisfy the title to the fullest and it will literally leave your children begging for more! Good luck cooking! Bon Appetite!

Who is this book for?

Dinners are made for sitting around the table and enjoying it! The recipe book here gives extremely simple recipes for possibly fussy kids.

This book is mainly for parents who have a hard time trying to coax their children into finishing their dinners and other meals! With these recipes below, parents will love cooking for their children and entire family, while the children will enjoy their meals even more. Soon enough you may actually have your child literally asking for a third and fourth serving! Picture that!

What will this book teach you?

This book is a great recipe book to flip through while sitting at a coffee shop or sitting at home and lazing around. More importantly, this book is great for parents to get a break from their regular cooking and try out something new.

This book will be able to teach you time management amongst learning new recipes. Try out these recipes more than once, and you will know which one takes time, and which doesn't and accordingly you can plan your meals for the week! This book will teach you to enjoy your time in the kitchen and to experiment with different ingredients at different times, so that no repetition is noticed.

1. Low Carb Pot Roast Swaddled in Bacon

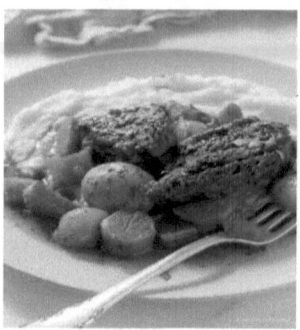

Summary

This beautiful delight made with bacon is an excellent dinner recipe for your family.

Ingredients

- 2-pound pork loin
- 1/2 pound very thinly sliced bacon
- 1 cup of white wine, dry is best
- 2 tablespoons of fresh rosemary, thinly chopped
- 1 tablespoon of olive oil
- Pinch of pepper
- Pinch of salt

Method

1. Start by moistening all sides of the roast with a pinch of salt and pepper. In a preheated oven, roast the pork and bacon for ten minutes. Dribble with olive oil and rosemary. Serve!

Use Rosemary in your Recipes

Not only does rosemary taste good, it is also packed with nutrients such as iron, calcium and Vitamin B6. Rosemary is highly rich in antioxidants. Rosemary is proven to have enhanced memory and concentration.

2. Cheesy Hot Tuna Melt Platter

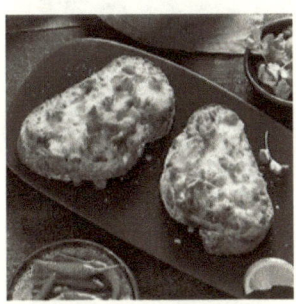

Summary

Another scrumptious recipe made with some cream and cheese to treat your taste buds!

Ingredients

- 1 can of white tuna in water, 6oz
- 1/4 cup of chopped up celery
- 1/4 cup of mayonnaise
- 1/3 cup sour cream
- 1 teaspoon of powdered mustard
- 1/2 teaspoon onion, powdered
- 1/4 teaspoon fresh thyme
- 1/4 teaspoon of fresh dill
- Pinch of salt
- 1/2 cup of favorite cheese, shredded
- 1/2 fresh tomato

Method

1. Except for the cheese and tomato, add all the ingredients to the tuna and stir. Then you have to microwave for 3 minutes. You are done!

Tuna is Good for You

It is advised that you eat fish at least once a week! It has high amounts of omega 3 which is good for you. It tastes great!

3. Seared Broccoli with a Lemon Twist

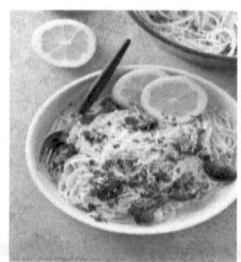

Summary

This recipe will make you fall in love with the leafy greens.

Ingredients

- 4 cups of fresh broccoli florets
- 1 tablespoon of olive oil
- 1/4 teaspoon of salt
- Ground pepper to taste
- Fresh lemon slices

Method

1. Preheat oven to 450° F. In a large mixing bowl, place broccoli florets and mix in oil with the salt and pepper. Roast in oven for 10 minutes before serving.

Health Benefits of Broccoli

Broccoli is packed with fiber and Vitamin C. It is an excellent way to prevent osteoarthritis. It is highly recommended for diabetic patients.

4. British Pork Cutlet Dressed in Cumberland Sauce

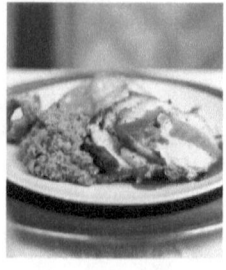

Summary

Prepared with the amazing Dijon Mustard, this pork recipe is an excellent variation to your menu list.

Ingredients

- 1 teaspoon virgin olive oil
- 2 thinly sliced boneless pork chops
- A dash of salt
- A dash of freshly ground pepper
- 1 small minced shallot
- 1/2 cup dry red wine
- 1/2 teaspoon cornstarch
- 1 1/2 teaspoons red-wine vinegar
- 1/2 teaspoon Dijon mustard

Method

1. Toss in all the ingredients together. In a saucepan heat olive oil on medium-high and cook the ingredients for 15 minutes. Viola! Serve!

Zucchini – The Delicious Vegetable You CANNOT Miss Out

Zucchini is rich in Vitamin C. The lutein in the vegetable promotes good eye sight. It has magnesium which promotes the healthy bone tissue development.

5. Savory Broccoli, Ginger and Sesame Stir Fry

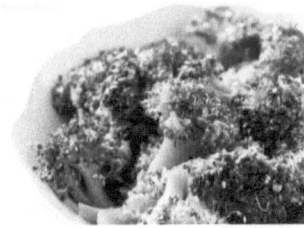

Summary

Cooked with sesame, this wondrous combination of ginger and sesame seeds is a classic recipe. Pair it with something meaty or eat it as it is, it is bound to taste as good as ever.

Ingredients

- 1 tablespoon sesame seeds
- 1/2 cup vegetable stock
- 1 tablespoon soy sauce
- 1 tablespoon dark sesame oil
- Drop of Canola oil
- 1 pound rinsed and dried broccoli florets
- 1 tablespoon of minced garlic
- 1 tablespoon minced ginger

Method

1. On the stove top warm a stick-free pan over medium heat; add sesame seeds, until brown. Toss in the rest of the ingredients. Dish out!

Sesame for the Health Conscious

Sesame seeds are an excellent source of copper. Sesame seeds also have a high content of calcium. With large contents of dietary fiber, this ingredient is a great remedy for avoiding constipation.

Read This FIRST - 100% FREE BONUS

FOR A LIMITED TIME ONLY – Get Olivia's best-selling book *"The #1 Cookbook: Over 170+ of the Most Popular Recipes Across 7 Different Cuisines!"* absolutely FREE!

Readers have absolutely loved this book because of the wide variety of recipes. It is highly recommended you check these recipes out and see what you can add to your home menu!

Once again, as a big thank-you for downloading this book, I'd like to offer it to you *100% FREE for a LIMITED TIME ONLY!*

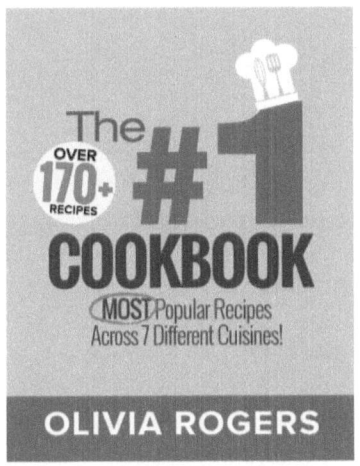

Get your free copy at:

TheMenuAtHome.com/Bonus

6. Monumental Meatloaf

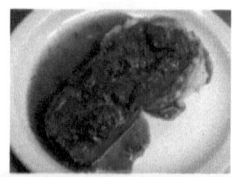

Summary

A meaty delight for all the meat lovers!

Ingredients

- 1 1/2 pounds of ground beef
- 1 1/4 teaspoon salt
- 1 egg
- Dash of pepper
- 1 cup bread crumbs
- 1/2 cup milk
- 1/3 cup ketchup
- 1 tablespoon onion powder

Method

1. Turn on and heat the oven to 350°F or 175°C. Mix all the ingredients and put the mixture in the prepared pan, making it fit to the sides of the pan. Place in oven for 1 hour. Once cooked, remove from the oven and let sit for 5 minutes.

You Should Eat Some Beef

It is high in protein. It is wholesome. It also has a lot of iron.

7. Aunt Sally's Savory Sausage Scramble

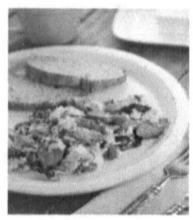

Summary

The Texan favorite, this sausage recipe is amazingly easy and delicious.

Ingredients

- 1/2 pound of lean breakfast sausage
- 1 1/2 cups of shredded potatoes
- 2 tablespoons of butter
- 6 oz. of shredded mild cheddar cheese
- 1/4 tablespoon of onion powder
- 16 oz. of cottage cheese
- 2 large eggs

Method

1. Turn on and preheat oven to 375°F or 190°C. Cook the sausage over medium heat until it is evenly brown on the outside. Then crumble. Mix all the other ingredients with crumbled sausage. Bake for 1 hour.

Incorporate Cheese

It is high in proteins. It is high in carbohydrates, so gives instant energy. It also has high content of calcium.

8. Mamma's Mushroom and Green Bean Mishmash

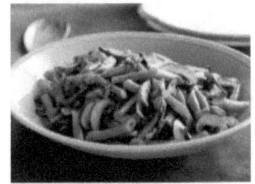

Summary

Another classic recipe, this will serve your craving taste buds just right! The beans used in the recipe fill you up nice and light! It is an overall well-balanced diet.

Ingredients

- 1/2 pound of fresh green beans
- 2 fresh carrots

- 1 sliced onion
- 1/2 pound of fresh mushrooms
- 1 teaspoon of seasoned salt
- 1/2 teaspoon of garlic powder

Method

1. Take a large frying pan and melt the butter over low to medium heat. Sauté the mushrooms adding the garlic powder to the pan. Once the mushrooms are almost tender add the beans, carrots and season salt to the pan. Cook for a final 5 minutes over low heat.

Benefits of Incorporating Beans into Your Life

Beans are an excellent alternatively to bread and pasta. It helps you maintain your weight. Beans are also high in proteins.

9. Mushroom Mayhem

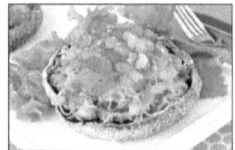

Summary

Next time when your kids are waiting for food on the table, making your life miserable, pick up this recipe and get done in 15 minutes!

Ingredients

- 12 whole fresh mushrooms
- 1 tablespoon Vegetable oil
- 1 tablespoon minced garlic
- 8 ounces of soft cream cheese
- 1/4 cup Parmesan cheese
- 1/4 teaspoon pepper

Method

1. Heat the oven to 350°F or 175°C. Toss in all the ingredients in a baking dish and bake for 15 minutes. Serve with garlic bread.

Health Benefits of Mushrooms

Mushrooms have selenium which is excellent for your bladder. Did you know that mushrooms produce Vitamin D when exposed to sunlight? Vitamin D helps the calcium absorb into your bones and prevent osteoporosis.

10. Spooky Pumpkin Seeds with Baked Chicken

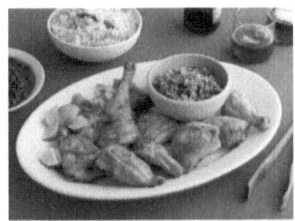

Summary

A unique combination, this new recipe will let you savor the goodness of pumpkin seeds and garlic powder. Paired with baked chicken, this recipe is satisfying for the belly as well as your taste buds!

Ingredients

- 1 1/2 tablespoon Margarine
- 1/2 teaspoon salt
- 1/8 teaspoon garlic powder
- 2 teaspoon Worcestershire sauce
- 2 cups whole pumpkin seeds

Method

1. Set oven to 275°F/135°C. Mix all the ingredients together and put the mixture in a shallow glass baking dish and bake for an hour. Serve with Baked chicken.

The Numerous Health Benefits of Pumpkin Seeds

Rich in minerals such as zinc, the WHO recommends a regular intake of the nutritious pumpkin seeds. Pumpkin seeds do not only provide us with Vitamin E, they provide us with Vitamin E in a wide diversity of forms. Did you know that the recommended time for roasting pumpkin seeds is no more than 20 minutes?

11. Tummy Tempting Tomato Salsa with Roast Beef

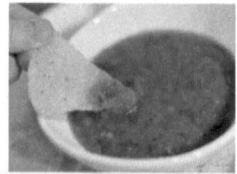

Summary

With controlled amount of calories, unlike the bottles of salsa you find in stores, this simple recipe will help you create a healthy sauce, ideal with roast beef. The lime juice used in the recipe adds to the tanginess of this exquisite recipe.

Ingredients

- 2 finely chopped fresh tomatoes
- 1/2 cup diced onion
- 5 minced serrano chilies
- 1/2 cup chopped cilantro
- 1 teaspoon salt
- 2 teaspoons Lime juice

Method

1. Simply mix all the ingredients together in a large bowl and let sit in the refrigerator for an hour before using. Serve with Roast beef.

The Good Tomatoes

They are high in Vitamins and minerals. They add color to your food. Did you know tomato is a fruit?

12. Happy Humming Hummus with Pita Bread

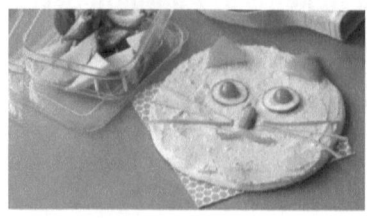

Summary

A classic favorite with the pita bread, this recipe offers a uniquely smooth texture.

Ingredients

- 1 clove of garlic
- 19 ounces or 1 can of garbanzo beans
- 4 tbsps. Lemon juice
- 2 tbsps. Tahini
- 1 teaspoon salt
- 1 tbsp. Olive oil

Method

1. Add to the blender; the chopped garlic, garbanzo beans, keeping a small tablespoon out to complete the dish later. Add the lemon juice, tahini, and salt. Blend until the mixture is creamy. Pour the mixture into a decorative serving bowl. Serve with pita bread.

Garbanzo Beans for the Healthy Low-Carb Diet Followers

Garbanzo beans have proven to be the favorite ingredient for those looking to lose weight. Studies have shown that individuals were more satisfied with their food, when garbanzo beans were included in the recipe! They help curb the craving you get in between your meals.

13. Texan Scramble

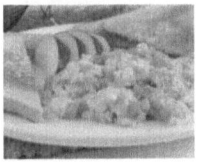

Summary

The delicious recipe makes use of the very healthy spinach to make the dish stand out.

Ingredients

- 5 eggs

- 2 tbsp. water
- 1/8 cup chopped green pepper
- 1/8 cup chopped red onion
- 2 cherry tomatoes, diced
- 1/2 cup frozen spinach, thawed and drained
- 5 jalapeno pepper slices, chopped
- 1 slice pepper jack cheese (or cheddar)
- 2 tbsp. Pace Salsa

Method

1. Use a pan or skillet with medium heat and add some oil. Mix all the ingredients (except cheese) together and throw them in. Add the cheese when the rest has reached the consistency you want. Turn off heat and let it sit for 3 minutes. Add some salsa and bacon/ beef strips.

Spinach Is for Strength

Like all green vegetables, spinach is very high vitamins and minerals. The antioxidants found in spinach help the body fight the cancerous growth. Spinach is highly recommended in appropriate dozes on a weekly basis.

14. Chicken Salad

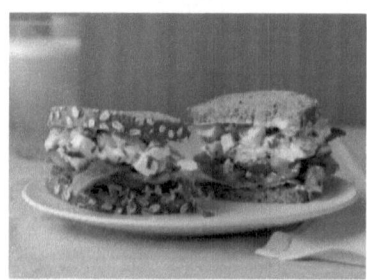

Summary

Sometimes to need to have something light for dinner!

Ingredients

- 1 boneless chicken breast, grilled
- 4 ounces leaf lettuce, chopped, about 2 cups
- 1/2 small tomato
- 1/2-ounce Swiss cheese, julienned

- 1-2 crisp pieces bacon, crumbled
- 1/2 hard-boiled egg, sliced in half
- 2 tablespoons Ranch dressing
- Dash pepper
- Pinch fresh parsley, chopped, optional

Method

1. Toss in all the ingredients. You're done!

Eggs for Your Health

Eggs are packed with protein and stimulate growth in the body. Did you know that 90% of the cholesterol in the egg is in the yolk? Those struggling with high cholesterol level are recommended to only use the white part of the egg.

15. Shrimp & Avocado Salad

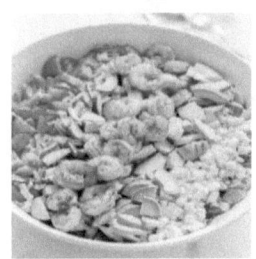

Summary

This is another light dinner recipe for a relaxing evening.

Ingredients

- Dressing of your choice
- 1 lb. cooked shrimps
- 2 ripe avocados
- 4 cups lettuce or baby greens

Method

1. Pour the dressing over the shrimp. Stir to coat. Cover and refrigerate for at least 1 hour. Toss it in with the Veggies and enjoy!

Health Benefits of Shrimp

Shrimps are recommended to be eaten at least every two weeks. Easy to cook and even easier to eat, this is an ideal food for kids and grown-ups. It is also packed with 52% protein and 31% iodine, which makes it especially healthy for kids.

16. Coconut Pancakes

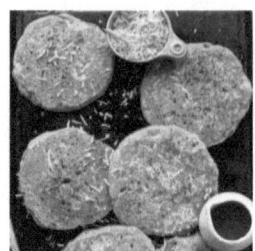

Summary

Who told you, you couldn't have pancakes for dinner? With the soothing aroma of the coconut, this coconut recipe is great for the kids and grown-ups alike.

Ingredients

- 2 large eggs
- 3 tablespoons full fat coconut milk
- 1/2 mashed ripe banana (about 2 tablespoons)
- 1/2 teaspoon apple cider vinegar
- 1/2 teaspoon vanilla extract
- 1 1/2 tablespoons of Bob's Red Mill organic coconut flour
- 1/2 teaspoon cinnamon
- 1/4 teaspoon baking soda
- 1 small pinch of salt
- coconut oil (for frying)

Method

1. Mix together eggs, coconut milk, mashed banana, apple cider vinegar, and vanilla extract and the rest of the ingredients. Put some butter in a pan and add a tablespoon of the mixture. Let it cook for around 30 seconds each side.

Coconut and Health

Coconut has proven to be a very common ingredient used in the households commonly; eat it raw, drink it up or prepare recipes like this, coconut, with all its health benefits, is a perfect pick! Very high in Vitamin A, coconuts are very good for the eyes! Coconuts are also used to stimulate hair and nail growth.

17. Shrimp, Leek, and Spinach Pasta

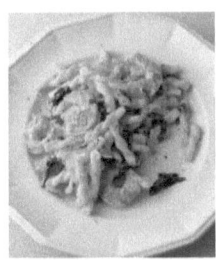

Summary

A unique combination of leek and shrimps, this recipe is there to please!

Ingredients

- 3/4-pound cooked pasta
- 2 tablespoons unsalted butter
- 2 leeks
- Salt and black pepper
- pound shrimp (sautéed)
- Zest of 1 lemon
- 3/4 cup heavy cream
- 10 ounces baby spinach

Method

1. Toss in all the ingredients and let it cook for 10 minutes (keep the pasta aside). Pour over pasta and enjoy!

Leeks and Benefits

Leeks are high in minerals and vitamins. It is not only very good for the eye sight, it also tastes great! These are also very low in calories and form the perfect ingredient of a diet conscious individual!

18. Spicy Salmon and Rice

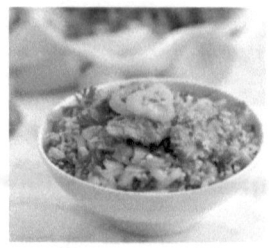

Summary

With a tinge of honey, this salmon recipe is sure to excite you!

Ingredients

- 2 tablespoons honey
- 1 tablespoon soy sauce
- 1/4 teaspoon crushed red pepper
- 4 6-ounce salmon fillets
- 1 cup rice (Cooked)

Method

1. Marinade the salmon with all the ingredients (Don't add the cooked rice of course!). Cook for 10 minutes in total. Serve with rice.

Honey for The Money!

Honey is the perfect antioxidant. Some people use it to cure diabetes! That's strange, right? Like the apple, honey is also said to keep the doctor away!

19. Chicken, Zucchini with Prosciutto

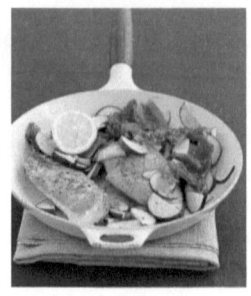

Summary

A unique combination, this savory recipe cooked in a total of 15 minutes will definitely take your taste buds on a joy ride!

Ingredients

- 4 boneless chicken breasts
- 2 tablespoons olive oil
- 1/4-pound prosciutto
- 3 small zucchinis, thinly sliced
- 1 clove garlic, sliced
- 1 lemon
- Salt and pepper to taste

Method

1. Marinate the chicken and the vegetables with all the ingredients. Toss it in the oven and let it bake for 15 minutes. You are done!

Why Prosciutto?

It is packed with protein. It enhances the taste of chicken. It also caters to the sodium requirement in the body.

20. Pecorino Chicken

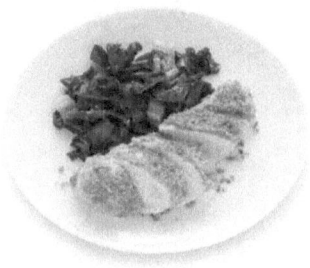

Summary

Write a little summary about why this dish is healthy and helps with the proposed solution. Maybe address one or two of the key ingredients.

Ingredients

- 5 slices sandwich bread
- 1/2 cup Grated pecorino
- 2 tablespoons butter
- Salt and black pepper to taste
- 4 pieces chicken breasts
- 1 tablespoon olive oil
- 2 bunches Swiss chard

Method

1. Blend all the ingredients, other than chicken and the chard, and coat the chicken with the blended mixture. Deep Fry. Sauté chard with salt and pepper and serve with chicken.

Cheers for the Chard!

Chard is an excellent source of Vitamin A, Vitamin K and C. Also, it is a great source of dietary fiber.

21. The Classic Chicken Curry

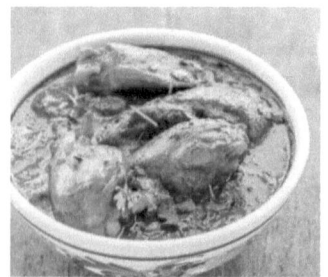

Summary

Write a little summary about why this dish is healthy and helps with the proposed solution. Maybe address one or two of the key ingredients.

Ingredients

- 1 cup white rice (cooked)
- An Ounce of steamed chicken breast, cubed into small pieces
- 1 tablespoon olive oil
- 1 small onion, sliced and browned

- 2 teaspoons curry powder
- 1/2 cup plain yogurt
- 3/4 cup heavy cream
- Fresh cilantro leaves, roughly chopped for garnish

Method

1. Keep the rice aside for serving. Put olive oil in a wok. Add the browned onions and the rest of the ingredients one by one. Add cream at the end. Serve with rice.

Health Benefits of Yogurt

It is an excellent source of calcium. It is high in protein. It is great for the skin!!

22. The Classic Grilled Cheese Sandwich

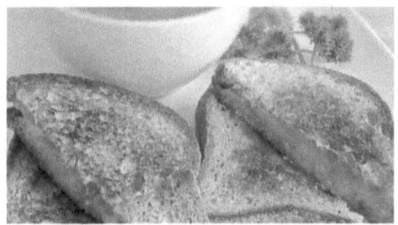

Summary

A quick, easy and simple fix made with cheddar cheese, this one is the kids' favorite.

Ingredients

- 1 thick slice of cheddar cheese
- 2 slices of bread
- Parsley for the garnish
- Oil for frying

Method

1. Sandwich the cheese in the middle of two slices of bread. Grill the sandwich on both sides until it turns golden on both sides and the cheese melts. Serve with garnished parsley.

Pick the Parsley

Packed with Vitamins and minerals, parsley not only adds flavor and color, it is very good for your body! Parsley can alternately be used for cilantro!

23. Slow Cooker Roast Chicken

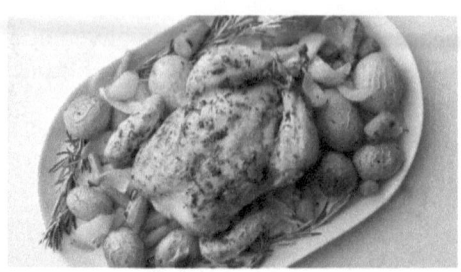

Summary

The easiest recipe to make, this chicken delight cooks itself in the cooker!

Ingredients

- 1 chicken boned-in
- Salt and pepper to taste
- 2 tbsp. soy sauce
- 1tbsp. olive oil

Method

1. Rub the chicken with salt, pepper, soy sauce and olive oil. Let it cook in the cooker for a good hour or until its done. Garnish with green chili and cilantro. Serve with rice.

Olive Oil for The Healthy

Olive oil is excellent for losing weight. Just replace the regular oil with olive oil in your diet and you will have made a great deal of difference. It is rich in Omega 3 and vitamins. It serves as an excellent salad dressing!

24. Barbequed Beef Sandwiches

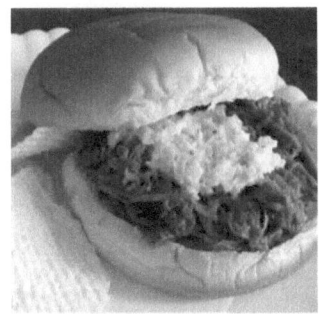

Summary

Best for kids, this is a basic recipe filled with exotic flavors. Made with a variety of breads, it is great for young and old alike!

Ingredients

- 1 lb. thinly sliced cooked roast beef, cut into 1-inch strips
- 6 hamburger buns, split
- Barbeque sauce

Method

1. Take the sandwich bread and grill on one side. Spread the barbeque sauce and beef and you are done! If you want you can add tomatoes and jalapeños to enhance the taste!

Whole Wheat Bread Instead of Normal Bread

It has essential fiber content that your body needs, unlike the white bread. It is packed with minerals. Also, it is more filling than white bread because it has more fiber.

25. Baked Spaghetti

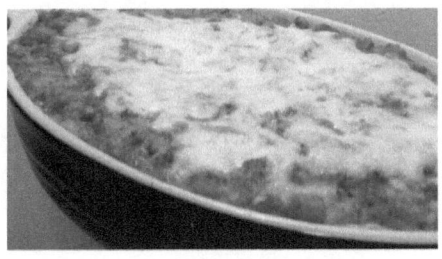

Summary

Another recipe for the kids, this recipe is exotic and colorful. Especially helpful for mothers when they looking to make something in no time.

Ingredients

- 1 package spaghetti, cooked
- 2 Tablespoons butter
- 1 cup grated Parmesan cheese
- 1 carton cottage cheese
- 1-pound ground beef
- 1 jar Italian-Style spaghetti sauce
- 1 package shredded mozzarella cheese

Method

1. Preheat oven to 400F. Cook spaghetti in melted butter over the stove. Arrange spaghetti in an oven prove dish. Layer it will cottage cheese and parmesan. Layer in the beef. Make the last layer of mozzarella. Bake for 15 minutes! Ta da! You're done!

Spaghettis!

It is an instant source of carbohydrates, so it best for the kids after their play session. Did you know spaghettis should be boiled whole, without breaking them into pieces? Something which so many people mistakenly do!

26. Pork Chops with Apples

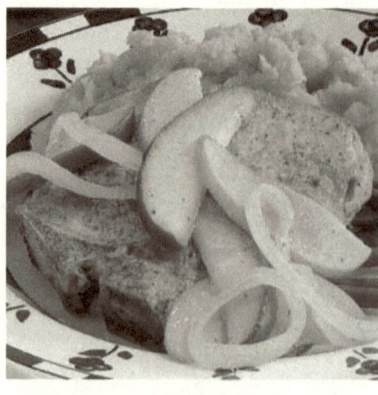

Summary

An exotic combination of apples and pork, this sweet and sour recipe will entice you and satiate your taste buds!

Ingredients

- 3-4 boned-in pork chops
- 2 Tablespoons oil
- 2 medium onions, thinly sliced
- 1 large green apple, cut into thin wedges
- 1 large red apple, cut into thin wedges
- 2 Tablespoons honey mustard
- 1 Tablespoon brown sugar
- Salt and pepper to taste

Method

1. Rub the chops with salt and pepper and cook on both sides until they turn golden on each side. Add the rest of the ingredients and sauté. Plate everything out and enjoy!

An Apple a Day Keeps the Doctor Away!

Apples are rich in iron! They have high levels of Vitamin A which makes them very good for the eyes! A perfect snack for a perfect day, apples are packed with healthy nutrition!

27. Red Potato Salad

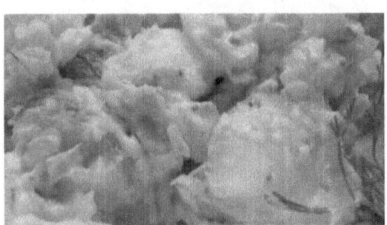

Summary

An easy recipe that can be eaten alone and if you want to pair it up with your favorite roasted recipe, go for it! With the simplest ingredients, this recipe is best for every day!

Ingredients

- 3 pounds unpeeled red potatoes boiled
- 4 eggs boiled and cubed
- 1 ½ cups mayonnaise
- 2 Tablespoons milk
- 2 Tablespoons distilled white vinegar
- ½ cup sliced green onions
- ½ teaspoon salt
- ¼ teaspoon ground black pepper
- 1 cup sliced celery

Method

1. Toss in everything together and you are done! For some extra seasoning, sprinkle some green onions on top.

Celery and Diet

With almost zero calories, this one is ideal for weight loss. Rich in mineral and vitamins, it is highly nutritious! Celery soup, especially, is excellent for losing weight.

28. Chili Coke Roast

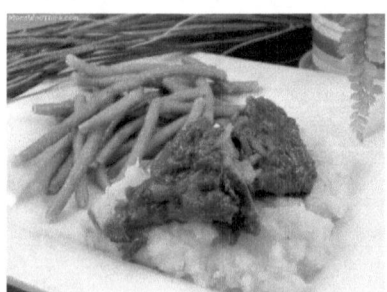

Summary

This simplistic recipe is perfect for a lazy evening. Packed with nutrients, this one is everyone's favorite!

Ingredients

- 1 beef roast (A three to Five Pound Piece should do just fine!)

- 1 can of Coca-Cola
- 1 package onion soup mix
- 1 bottle chili sauce

Method

1. Marinate the beef in all the ingredients mentioned. Cook for 7 to 8 hours in a crock pot! It's done. Plate out and enjoy!

Onions in Cooking!

Photo chemicals in onions help in the better functioning of Vitamin C in the body! An essential salad component, this is an everyday ingredient, that has long been used to treat inflammations and to heal infections.

29. Chicken Stroganoff

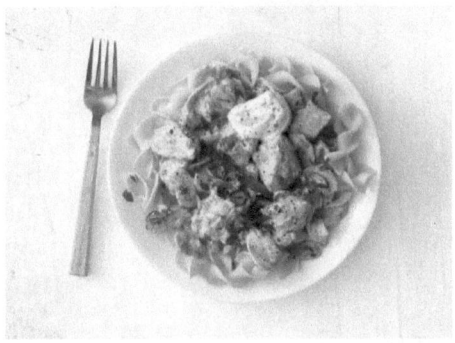

Summary

A classic recipe, this one is sure to leave the table even before it reaches it! Made with sour cream and egg noodles, this one is classically tasty!

Ingredients

- 2 Tablespoons butter
- 1 lb. chicken breast cut in strips
- 2 cups mushrooms
- 1 medium onion, chopped
- 1 can cream of chicken soup
- 1/2 cup sour cream
- 4 cups egg noodles

Method

1. Cook chicken in 1 Tablespoon butter. After it is tender, remove from stove. Cook the onions and mushrooms in remaining butter. Stir in soup and sour cream. Add everything together. Serve over noodles.

Mushroom and the Health Benefits

Mushrooms are high in anti-oxidants. They have a very low-calorie count, so they account for as an excellent ingredient for those who want to lose weight. And also, tasty as ever!

30. Lamb Chops and Peppercorns

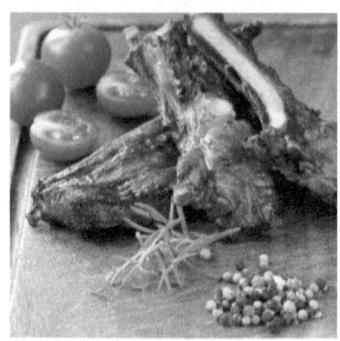

Summary

It's time to try some lamb in the kitchen! This exotic dinner recipe will encourage many complements for the chef! As easy as it is delicious, made with peppercorns, this recipe looks good too!

Ingredients

- 8 lamb loin chops
- 1/2 teaspoon cracked whole black peppercorns
- 1/2 teaspoon whole green peppercorns, crushed
- 1/2 teaspoon ground white pepper
- 1/2 cup dry red wine
- 1/4 cup olive oil
- 1-1/2 teaspoons snipped fresh rosemary
- 2 cloves grated garlic
- 1 Tablespoon Dijon-style mustard

Method

1. Marinade the lamb with all the ingredients. Don't add the peppers, we will keep them separate. Marinade the lamb in the fridge for about six hours.

2. Roast the lamb in the oven, using the broiler section for 3-4 minutes on each side. Roast the pepper with seasons or simply sauté the peppers. Dish out!

Peppers are Good for You!

Peppers are rich in Vitamin A and therefore, really good for your eyes! Did you know that they also support night vision? If you are looking to lose weight, peppers, especially red ones, are for you!

31. Roasted Chicken with Honey Glazed Sweet Potatoes

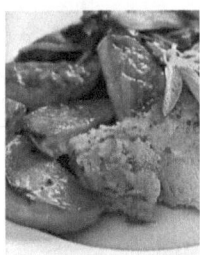

Summary

The chicken and sweet potato provide a delicious combination of protein, fiber, and tons of essential vitamins.

Ingredients

- 4 whole Chicken Thighs
- 2 lbs. Sweet Potatoes (peeled, sliced)
- 1 Habanero Chili (minced)
- ½ cup Chopped Onion
- 4 cloves Garlic (chopped)
- 3 Tbsps. Apple Cider Vinegar
- 4 Tbsps. Honey
- 2 Tbsps. Olive Oil
- 1 Tbsp. Allspice Berries (ground)
- 1 Tbsp. Fresh Ginger (peeled, chopped)

- 1 ½ tsp Fresh Thyme (chopped)
- 1 tsp Salt
- 1 tsp Black Pepper
- 1 tsp Cinnamon
- ¼ tsp Nutmeg
- 2 Tbsps. Butter (melted)
- 1 Tbsp. Fresh Squeezed Lime Juice
- Mango Chutney

Method

1. In a processor, pulse together the apple cider vinegar, garlic, onion, allspice, thyme, ginger, chili, cinnamon, nutmeg, salt, and black pepper. Blend until pureed. Place the chicken in a large zip lock bag. Add the marinade and seal. Turn and shake the bag gently to fully coat the chicken. Refrigerate overnight.

2. Preheat oven to 400° F. Place the chicken on a baking dish. Drizzle the marinade over it. Brush with olive oil. Bake for 45 minutes or until cooked through. For the sweet potatoes: whisk together honey, butter, lime juice, and cinnamon in a large bowl. Add slices of potato. Toss until coated.

3. Arrange the slices on a greased baking sheet in a single layer. Bake them with the chicken until tender (about 25 minutes). Serve with mango chutney on the side.

Fun Facts

Here are 3 reasons you should be eating more sweet potatoes: They have a richer flavor but nearly half the carbs of regular potatoes. They are high in fiber and Vitamin A. Sweet potatoes are great for your skin, adding a youthful glow.

32. Mushroom Potato Gratin

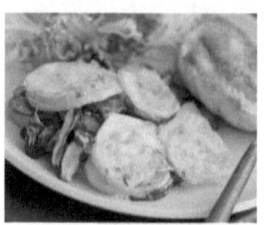

Summary

A hearty serving of mushroom and potato provides you with a good helping of key essential nutrients.

Ingredients

- 2 ½ lbs. Potatoes (peeled, thinly sliced)
- 12 oz. Crimini Mushrooms (sliced)
- 6 cloves Garlic (thinly sliced)
- 1 cup grated Parmesan Cheese
- 1 ¼ cup Heavy Whipping Cream
- 5 Tbsp. Olive Oil
- 2 Tbsp. Fresh Thyme (chopped)
- 1 ½ tsp Salt
- ¾ tsp Black Pepper

Method

1. Preheat oven to 375° F (unless freezing). Grease a baking dish with 2 tablespoons olive oil. Add a layer of sliced potatoes and sprinkle with salt and pepper. Pour 1/3 cup cream over the potatoes. Sprinkle with ¼ cup parmesan. Continue layering the ingredients in this way. Sprinkle thyme and garlic over the top. Bake for about 45 minutes or until potatoes are tender.

2. Toss mushrooms in a bowl with oil, salt, and pepper. Pour a ¼ cup cream and ¼ cup cheese over the top. Bake for another 20 minutes or until the edges start to turn gold and the mushrooms are tender. To reheat, cover in foil to prevent drying.

Tips

Use turnips in place of the potatoes if you are carb conscious. Add chicken or tuna for additional protein. Experiment with different sharp cheeses to land on your favorite flavor combination.

33. Meatball Mash

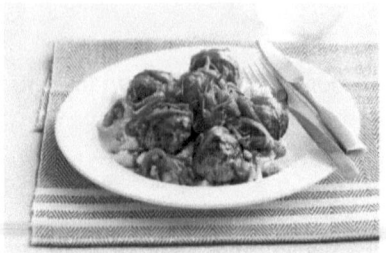

Summary

This takes the classic "meat and potatoes" to a delicious new level.

Ingredients

- 1 lbs. Ground Beef
- ½ cup Brown Rice
- 1 ½ cup Water
- 3-4 large Potatoes
- ½ cup Onion (chopped)
- 1 (15 oz.) can Tomato Sauce
- 2 ½ tsp Salt
- 1 clove Garlic (minced)
- 1 tsp Black Pepper
- 1 Egg
- ¼ cup Heavy Cream (or Buttermilk)
- 2-3 Tbsps. Butter
- 1 tsp Thyme
- 1 tsp Oregano

Method

1. Preheat oven to 350° F (unless freezing). Toss together ground beef, rice, onion, and ½ cup water in a large bowl. Add salt, pepper, garlic, and celery salt. Mix thoroughly.

2. Form 1 to 2-inch balls with the meat. In a large skillet, brown the meatballs and drain the fat. Combine tomato sauce and 1 cup water in a baking dish. Place the meatballs in the dish and roll to coat them in the tomato sauce. Cover and bake for about 45 minutes or until cooked through.

Tips

The rich flavor of this dish disguises the high nutrition value, making it the perfect dish for picky eaters. It's even better when served with a fresh salad on the side. Add 1 cup of rolled oats to the meat to add more fiber.

34. Smoked Turkey with Almond Mole

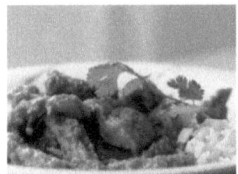

Summary

This dish is full of bold flavors that will make it hard to believe how amazingly nutritious it really is.

Ingredients

- 3 cups chopped Turkey Breast (cooked)
- ½ cup Roasted Almonds
- 1 (14.5 oz.) can Vegetable Broth
- 2 small Corn Tortillas (torn into bite sized pieces)
- 1 ½ cups Tomatoes (preferably fire-roasted, crushed)
- 1 (7 oz.) can Chiles in adobo sauce
- 2 dried Chiles (hot)
- 1 cup Onion (chopped)
- 2-3 cloves Garlic (minced)
- ½ tsp Olive Oil
- 1 Tbsp. Sugar
- 1 Tbsp. White Wine Vinegar
- 1/8 tsp Cloves (ground)
- ½ tsp Cumin
- ¼ tsp Salt

Method

1. Pulse almonds in a food processor until smooth. Set aside. In a large skillet, heat oil. Add chilies and sauté for 1-2 minutes. Add garlic and onion. Sauté for about 4 minutes. Add 1 canned chili. Leave it whole.

2. Add the tomatoes, broth, sugar, cloves, cumin, and salt. Bring to a boil. Reduce heat and simmer for 15 minutes. Remove from heat and use a stick blender to blend until smooth (or spoon into the food processor). Return to heat. Add ground almonds and vinegar. Cook for 1-2 minutes. Stir in cooked turkey.

Tips

Use chicken or other poultry instead of turkey if not available. Add more or fewer chilies to taste. Use almond meal instead of whole almonds to save yourself a step.

35. Stuffed Chicken Rolls

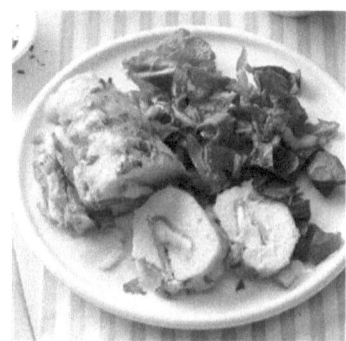

Summary

Melted cheese and crunchy bread crumbs create bold combinations of texture in this dish.

Ingredients

- 4 Chicken Breasts (skinless, boneless)
- 1 cup Bread Crumbs (seasoned)
- ½ cup Parmesan Cheese (grated)
- ¼ cup Butter (melted)
- 1 (8 oz.) package Cream Cheese
- 2-3 cloves Garlic (minced)

Method

1. Preheat oven to 350° F (unless freezing). Pound chicken until thinned. In a bowl, combine bread crumbs and cheese. Dip one side of each

breast into the melted butter. Immediately dip the same side into the bread crumb and cheese mixture.

2. On the clean side of the breast, place 1-2 dollops of cream cheese. Roll them so that the cream cheese is on the inside. Secure with a toothpick. Bake for 40 minutes or until cooked through.

Tips

The melted cheese and crunchy bread crumbs make this the perfect dish for disguising a serving of veggies. Add carrot, spinach, or asparagus to the filing. Replace half the butter with olive oil for a healthier fat. Serve on a bed of brown rice or quinoa for added fiber.

36. Juicy Make Ahead Ribs

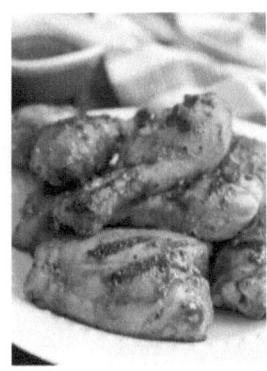

Summary

Prepare this simple yet irresistibly scrumptious sauce and leave your ribs to marinate overnight in the fridge. Drizzle the rest over some rice!

Ingredients

- 4 lbs. Pork Spareribs
- ½ cup Honey
- ¼ cup Soy Sauce
- ¼ cup White Vinegar
- 3 cloves Garlic (minced)
- 2 Tbsps. Sugar
- 1 Tbsps. Molasses
- 1 tsp Baking Soda

Method

1. Preheat oven to 375° F (unless freezing). Cut up the ribs into single pieces. In a separate bowl, combine soy sauce, vinegar, honey, sugar, molasses, and garlic. Blend thoroughly. Add baking soda and stir until it begins to foam. Dip the ribs into the bowl and coat thoroughly (until dripping with sauce).

2. Cover a baking sheet with foil and arrange the ribs in a single layer. Pour the remaining sauce over the top of the ribs. Cover with another layer of foil and bake for 1 hour or until cooked through.

Tips

Serve with a fresh salad or a side of quinoa to add more nutrition value. Keep these ready-to-go ribs on hand for spontaneous barbecues or dinner parties. Use low sodium soy sauce to keep your salt intake down.

37. Stuffed Lasagna Rolls

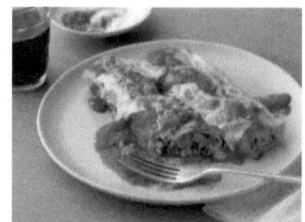

Summary

These single serving style lasagna rolls are easy, versatile, and perfect to freeze for lunches and dinners throughout the week.

Ingredients

- 1 (16 oz.) package Lasagna Noodles
- 1 (10 oz.) package Spinach (frozen, chopped)
- 1 lbs. Mozzarella (shredded)
- 1 (15 oz.) package Ricotta
- 2 cups Parmesan (grated)
- 1 lbs. Tofu (firm)
- 1 (28 oz.) jar Pasta Sauce (your favorite kind)

Method

1. Bring a large pot of water to a boil. Add lasagna noodles and cook until slightly underdone (about 5-8 minutes). Drain and rinse. Mix together mozzarella, parmesan, ricotta, tofu, and spinach in a large mixing bowl.

2. Lay a noodle flat. Spread a layer of cheese mixture across it. Then spread a layer of sauce on top of that. Roll the noodle up and place it in a baking dish (with the seam side down). Repeat this for all lasagna noodles. Drizzle extra sauce over the top and grate a little extra parmesan over as well. Bake for about 30 minutes at 350° F (until bubbling).

Tips

Replace the tofu with squash, turnip, or sweet potato for more flavor. Serve with a fresh salad or a side of quinoa. Pair with a glass of red wine to boost heart health.

38. Prosciutto Wrapped Chicken with Pesto Pasta

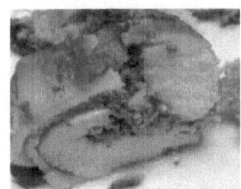

Summary

This delicious and healthy dish is sure to impress even the pickiest of eaters. It's the perfect dish to come home to after a long day of work.

Ingredients

- 4 Chicken Breasts (skinless, boneless)
- 4 slices Prosciutto (large, thin)
- ¾ cup Goat Cheese (soft)
- 2 Shallots (chopped)
- 2 cloves Garlic (minced)
- 3 Dates (chopped)
- 1 Tbsp. Basil
- 3 large handfuls Fresh Basil

- 1 handful Pine Nuts
- 1 handful Parmesan Cheese (grated)
- 1 tsp Thyme
- Salt
- ¼ tsp Black Pepper
- Fresh Lemon Juice
- 1 (16 oz.) package Whole Grain Linguine

Method

1. In a food processor, combine 1 clove garlic, pine nuts, fresh basil, and a pinch of salt. Pour mixture into a bowl. Add parmesan and a little olive oil. Add just enough oil to create a gooey consistency. Add a squeeze of lemon juice. Set aside.

2. Grease a baking sheet with olive oil (unless freezing). Set aside. Heat 1 tablespoon olive oil in a pan on medium heat. Add shallots. Cook for about 3 minutes. Add thyme, salt, pepper, and garlic. Cook for 2 minutes. Pour this mixture into a bowl. Add goat cheese, basil, and dates. Mix well.

3. Slice a 1" slit into the thick side of each breast. Use your fingers to expand this into a deep pocket. Stuff each pocket with the cheese and shallot mixture (about ¼ cup per breast). Wrap each breast in a slice of prosciutto. Place them on the baking sheet (seam side down). Bake for about 40 minutes at 350° F or until prosciutto is crispy and browned.

Fun Facts

Each ingredient in this recipe packs a nutritious punch. It's the ideal balance of protein, fiber, and unsaturated fats. Basil is a natural remedy for upset stomachs and bad breath. Goat cheese is one of the few animal products that contains vitamin C.

39. Make Ahead Pierogies

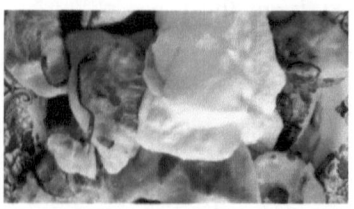

Summary

Pierogies are wonderfully simple and extremely versatile. Modify this recipe to your own tastes.

Ingredients

- 3 cups Whole Grain Flour
- 2 cups Mashed Potatoes (cold)
- 1 (16oz.) package Sour Cream
- ½ cup Butter
- 2 large Onions (chopped)

Method

1. In a large mixing bowl, add sour cream and flour. Blend until it forms a dough. Roll the dough out on a floured surface until very thin. Cut out 3 ½" circles. Add about a teaspoon of mashed potato to the center of each dough circle. Fold the circle in half and press the edges with a fork. Set aside under a towel.

2. Bring a large pot of water to a boil. Add the pierogies to the water a few at a time. Let them boil for about 4 minutes. Remove gently. Melt butter in a pan on medium low heat. Add onions and cook for about 4-5 minutes. Add pierogies and cook about 3 minutes (until browned on the bottom).

Tips

Don't be afraid to experiment. Try any filling you can think of from sweet to savory and everything in between. Serve these on a bed of fresh salad for added texture and fiber. Use mashed turnip instead of potato for a lower carb alternative.

40. Almond Crusted Chicken Casserole

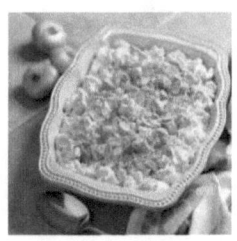

Summary

This simple casserole dish is a complete meal on its own.

Ingredients

- 5 cups Chicken (diced, cooked)
- 1 ½ cups Quinoa
- 3 cups Water
- 1 ½ cups Almonds (sliced)
- 1 cup Celery (chopped)
- 3 cups Cornflakes
- ½ cup Mayonnaise
- ½ cup Greek Yogurt (plain)
- 1 (10 oz.) can Cream of Mushroom Soup (condensed)
- 2 cups Chicken Broth
- 2 Tbsps. Lemon Juice
- 3 Tbsps. Onion (chopped)
- 1 (8 oz.) can Water Chestnuts
- 1 cup Butter (melted)
- 2 tsp White Pepper
- 1 Tbsp. Salt

Method

1. In a pot, combine quinoa and water. Bring to a boil. Reduce heat to low, cover, and simmer until the water is completely absorbed and quinoa is fluffy. Grease a baking dish. Set aside. In a large bowl, mix quinoa, chicken, yogurt, mayonnaise, cream of mushroom soup, and broth. Add lemon juice, water chestnuts, onion, and 1 cup sliced almonds. Season with salt and pepper to taste. Pour mixture into baking dish.

2. In another bowl, mix the rest of the almonds, cornflakes, and melted butter. Spread on top of the casserole. Bake for 40 minutes at 350° F or until browned and crispy.

Fun Facts

The almonds are rich in vitamin E which is great for your skin and hair. Greek yogurt is full of probiotics which helps improve digestion. The high fiber content in this dish also helps digestion and detoxes your skin.

41. Make Ahead Quiche

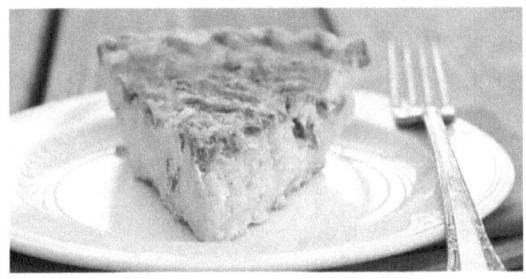

Summary

Quiche makes a perfect breakfast, lunch, or dinner. You can easily modify it to your own tastes.

Ingredients

- 1 (9") raw Pie Crust
- 1 ½ cups Swiss Cheese (shredded)
- ½ cup Ham (diced, cooked)
- 1 cup Milk
- 3 Eggs
- 4 tsp Whole Grain Flour
- ¼ tsp Salt
- ¼ tsp Dry Mustard (ground)

Method

1. In a bowl, combine flour and cheese. Spread this mixture across the bottom of your pie crust. Sprinkle in the ham. In another bowl, mix milk, cream, and eggs together. Add salt and mustard powder. Beat until thoroughly combined. Pour into the pie crust. Cover the crust in foil to prevent burning. Bake for about 1 hour at 400° F or until the filling sets.

Fun Facts

Despite the bad reputation, eggs actually lower bad cholesterol. Eggs are a superfood with a full range of nutrients in one tiny shell. Steep the egg shells in water for a day before watering flowers to provide essential minerals and nutrients to plants.

42. Sausage Manicotti

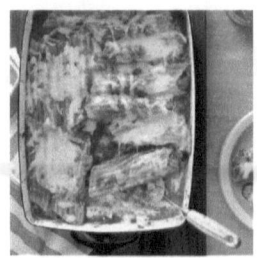

Summary

This hearty dish is simple and quick. It pairs well with a fresh salad and a glass of red wine.

Ingredients

- 10 Manicotti Shells
- 1 lbs. Turkey Italian Sausage
- 1 cup Green Bell Pepper (chopped)
- 1 ½ cups Onion (chopped)
- 2 cups Milk
- 2 cups Tomato Sauce (with Basil)
- ¼ cup Parmesan Cheese (grated)
- 1 ½ cups Mozzarella (shredded)
- 1 tsp Black Pepper
- 2 Tbsps. Whole Grain Flour
- 2 Tbsps. Butter (plus more for greasing)

Method

1. Boil manicotti shells until just underdone. Heat oil in a pan over medium high heat. Remove sausage from casing and add to pan. Crumble the sausage and stir until browned (about 5 minutes). Add onion and bell pepper. Cook about 5 minutes.

2. In a pot, melt butter over medium heat. Add flour. Cook 2 minutes, whisking constantly. Remove from heat and add milk while stirring with a whisk. Return to heat and bring to a boil. Cook until thickened (About 6 minutes), whisking constantly. Remove from heat. Stir in black pepper. Pour ½ cup of this mixture into the sausage mix. Stir well.

3. Spoon 1/3 cup of this mixture into each manicotti shell. Place manicotti on a greased baking dish. Pour remaining milk mixture over the manicotti shells. Sprinkle the mozzarella over the surface. Spread a layer of tomato sauce. Sprinkle parmesan cheese. Bake for 35 minutes at 350° F (or until bubbly).

Tips

Use shredded chicken as a substitute for turkey sausage for a different texture. Try different veggie combinations to keep this dish fresh and new. Replace ½ cup mozzarella with ricotta for a lighter, fluffier filling.

43. Onion Pepper Sausage Calzone

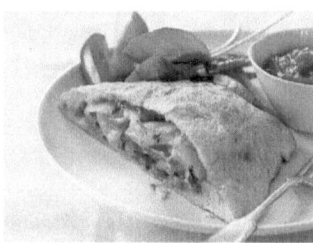

Summary

This highly versatile and surprisingly nutritious recipe can also be used for pizzas.

Ingredients

- 2 ¼ cups Whole Grain Flour
- ½ package Active Dry Yeast (about 1 1/8 tsp)
- ½ cup Warm Water
- ¾ cup Cold Water
- 2 Tbsps. Olive Oil
- 1 tsp Sugar
- 1 tsp Salt
- 1 lbs. Turkey Italian Sausage
- 1 large Onion (sliced)
- 1 Red Bell Pepper (sliced)
- 1 Yellow Bell Pepper (sliced)
- 1 ¾ cups Pizza Sauce
- 1 1/3 cups Mozzarella (shredded)

Method

1. Dissolve the yeast in warm water for 5 minutes. In a separate bowl, whisk together sugar, salt, oil, and cold water. Add yeast mixture. Add flour 1 cup at a time. Mix thoroughly until it begins to form into a smooth ball.

2. Turn dough onto floured surface and knead for 5 minutes (dough should be smooth but still slightly sticky). Divide the dough into 4 equal pieces. Roll each piece out in a rectangle (approximately 9" x 5"). Spread a layer of sauce over each piece. Leave a ½" border on all sides. Arrange sausage, onion, and bell pepper evenly on all pieces. Sprinkle cheese over the tops. Fold the dough over lengthwise. Press the edges down with a fork. Bake for about 15 minutes at 500° F or until golden brown.

Tips

Prepare and freeze the dough in large quantities for spontaneous pizza or calzone nights. Stuff lots of different veggies into your calzone to make sure you are getting all your veggies for the day.

44. Hearty Chicken & Noodle Soup

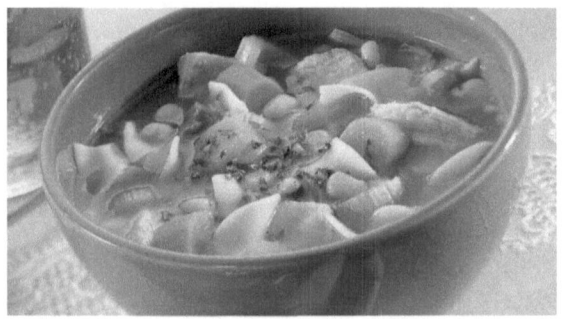

Summary

This rich soup is easy to prepare and soothes the soul.

Ingredients

- 1 lbs. Beans (canned, borlotti or pinto)
- 1 lbs. Chicken Breast (cubed)
- 7 cups Chicken Broth

- 2 medium Onions (chopped)
- 2 medium Carrots (chopped)
- 2 stalks Celery (chopped)
- 5 cloves Garlic (minced)
- ¾ lbs. Pasta (preferably macaroni, penne, or other tube-shaped pasta)
- 1 tsp Black Pepper
- 1 tsp Rosemary
- 1 tsp Thyme

Method

1. In a large pot, combine chicken and broth. Bring to a boil. Reduce heat to medium, add carrots, onion, and celery. Let simmer for 15 minutes. Add pepper, rosemary, thyme, garlic, and pasta. Let simmer another 10 minutes or until pasta is cooked.

Fun Facts

Beans are an amazing source of protein, fiber, and minerals. It should be a staple of any healthy diet. Garlic is a natural remedy for the common cold, flu, and other viral or bacterial infections. The beta carotene found in carrots helps protect your skin from sun damage and improves eye health.

45. Beef & Barley Soup

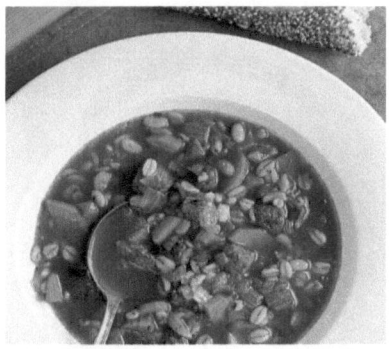

Summary

This rich and flavorful soup is perfect for fall or winter.

Ingredients

- 1.5 oz. Mushrooms (dried, chopped)

- 1 lbs. Beef (cross cut)
- 8 cups Water
- 1 large Onion (chopped)
- 2 large Carrots (quartered)
- 2 stalks Celery (cut into 1" slices)
- ½ cup Pearl Barley
- 2 ½ tsp Salt
- ½ tsp Black Pepper

Method

1. In a large pot, combine beef and water. Bring to a boil. Reduce heat to a simmer and leave it for 1 hour or until the meat is tender. Discard bones, fat, and gristle. Cut meat into bite-size pieces. Return meet to water. Add mushrooms, onions, carrots, celery, barley, salt and pepper. Let simmer for about 40 minutes or until barley is tender.

Fun Facts

Barley is a great source of most vitamins and minerals. This soup is a perfect way to eat healthy on a budget. Carrots are actually more nutritious when cooked because your body can digest the vitamins more easily.

46. Mushroom Soup with Herbed Cream

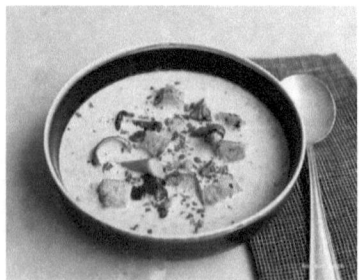

Summary

This exquisite soup tastes like a 5-star restaurant recipe but is surprisingly simple to make.

Ingredients

- 2 lbs. Mushrooms (quartered)
- 3 large Leeks (diced)

- 6 cups Chicken Stock
- 6 Tbsps. Butter
- ½ cup Heavy Cream
- 6 Tbsps. Whole Grain Flour
- 3 tsp Thyme
- 1 ½ tsp Salt
- ¾ tsp Black Pepper

Method

1. Use an electric mixer to beat cream until it forms soft peaks. Add 2 teaspoons thyme and continue mixing. Cover and set in the fridge (between 2 to 24 hours).

2. In a large pot, heat 2 tablespoons butter. Add 1 lbs. mushrooms. Cook until lightly browned. Transfer to a large bowl. Repeat this process for the remaining mushrooms. Heat 2 tablespoons butter in the same pot. Add leeks. Cover and cook until soft (about 5 minutes). Stir often. Add mushrooms. Sprinkle in flour. Stir until well mixed.

3. Add chicken stock, salt, pepper, and 1 teaspoon thyme. Bring to a boil. Reduce to heat to low and let simmer 20 minutes with lid halfway on. When serving, add a dollop of herbed cream to each bowl.

Fun Facts

Mushrooms are the only natural source of vitamin D aside from the sun (everything else is fortified). Multiple studies have found that mushrooms boost your immune system. Mushrooms are a great source of antioxidants.

47. Cozy Butternut Squash Soup

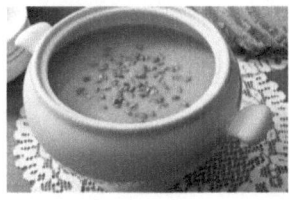

Summary

The full-bodied flavor of butternut squash is celebrated in this dish.

Ingredients

- 4 cups Butternut Squash (cubed)
- 1 cup Chicken Broth
- 1 (14 oz.) can Coconut Milk
- ½ cup Roasted Peanuts (unsalted)
- 1 cup Onion (chopped)
- 2 ½ tsp Red Curry Paste
- 1 clove Garlic (minced)
- 1 tsp Fresh Ginger (minced)
- 2 tsp Brown Sugar
- 1 ½ tsp Fish Sauce
- ¼ tsp Salt

Method

1. In a large pot, bring broth and squash to a boil. Reduce heat to medium and let simmer for 20 minutes (or until squash is tender). Add coconut milk, brown sugar, fish sauce, and salt. Let simmer another 10 minutes.

2. Heat oil in a pan on medium-high heat. Add onion. Cook 3 minutes. Add curry paste, ginger, and garlic. Cook 1 minute, stirring constantly. Add curry paste mixture to the pot. Let simmer 10 minutes. Remove from heat. Use a stick blender (or food processor) to blend the soup until smooth. Spoon into serving bowls. Top with peanuts.

Tips

If you want to save time on this recipe, buy frozen pureed butternut squash. You'll need 2 12oz. packages. Roast the seeds in honey and salt for a scrumptious snack. Serve this dish with brown rice or quinoa for added fiber.

48. Herbed Pork & Beans

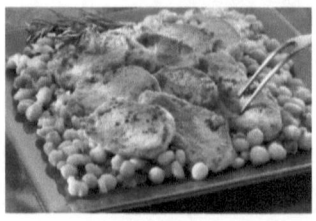

Summary

This variation on a classic will spice up your weekly menu.

Ingredients

- 1 cup White Beans
- 1 lbs. Pork Roast (boneless, cubed)
- 2 cups Chicken Broth
- 6 cloves Garlic (chopped)
- 2 cups Onion (chopped)
- ½ cup Water
- ½ cup Carrot (chopped)
- 1 tsp Sage
- 2 tsp Thyme
- ½ tsp Black Pepper
- ½ tsp Salt

Method

1. Heat 1 tablespoon oil in a pan. Sprinkle salt and pepper over the pork. Add to pan. Cook 6 minutes (brown all sides). Add beans, broth, sage, thyme, onion, carrot. Bring to a boil then reduce to medium low, cover, and let simmer 40 minutes. Add garlic. Let simmer another 20 minutes.

Tips

Enrich the flavor by doing the beans from scratch. Put 1 cup of dry beans in a crock pot with 6 cups water and let it cook at a low temperature while you're at work. Use chicken instead of pork for a lighter option. Soak up the broth with a slice of whole grain bread.

49. Green Chili

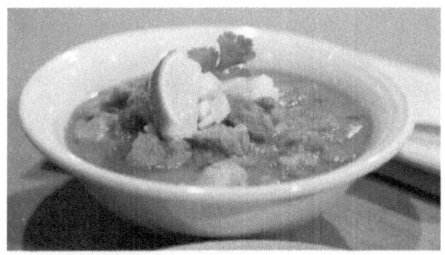

Summary

Add a little heat to your menu with this delicious chili.

Ingredients

- 1 lbs. Chicken Breasts (boneless, skinless, cubed)
- 1 ½ cups Onion (chopped)
- ¼ cup Sharp Cheddar (shredded)
- 1 (15 oz.) can Kidney Beans
- 1 (15 oz.) can Tomatoes
- 1 (4 oz.) can Diced Green Chilies
- 1 medium Green Onion (sliced)
- ½ cup Salsa Verde
- 1 (12 oz.) bottle Dark Beer
- 5 cloves Garlic (minced)
- 1 Tbsp. Olive Oil
- 1 Tbsp. Chili Powder
- 1 tsp Hot Paprika

Method

1. Heat oil in a pan over medium-high heat. Add chicken. Cook until no longer pink. Add onion, paprika, and chili powder. Cook 4 minutes. Add garlic. Cook 1 minute.

2. Add beer. Bring to a boil. Cook until liquid is almost evaporated. Add salsa, beans, tomatoes, chilies. Reduce heat. Let simmer 30 minutes. Stir occasionally. Ladle into bowls and top with cheese and green onion.

Fun Facts

Here's 3 reasons to embrace spicy foods: Capsaicin (the ingredient that gives chilies their heat) boosts your metabolism, helping you lose weight. Capsaicin may reduce your risk of heart attack and disease. Some studies show it may even help fight cancer!

50. Rich & Hearty Pork Stew

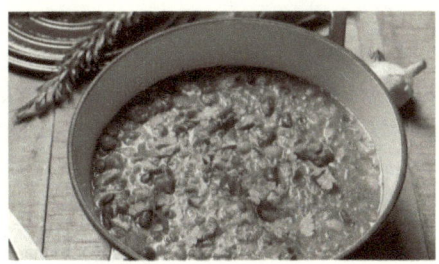

Summary

This stew will warm you up while providing multiple servings of almost every food group.

Ingredients

- 1 ½ lbs. Pork Tenderloin (trimmed, cubed)
- 1 (28 oz.) can Hominy
- 2 ½ cups Chicken Broth
- 1 (14.5 oz.) can Fire Roasted Tomatoes (diced)
- 1 ½ cups Green Bell Pepper (chopped)
- 2 cups Onion (chopped)
- 1-2 cloves Garlic (minced)
- 1 Tbsp. Olive Oil
- 2 Tbsp. Chili Powder
- 2 tsp Oregano
- 1 ½ tsp Smoked Paprika
- ½ tsp Salt
- 1 tsp Cumin

Method

1. In a large bowl, mix cumin, paprika, oregano, chili powder, and salt. Remove 1 ½ teaspoons of spice mixture. Set aside. Add pork to the bowl. Toss to coat.

2. Heat oil in a large pot over medium-high heat. Add pork and spice mixture. Cook until browned. Remove pork. Set aside. Add a little more oil. Add onion, bell pepper, and garlic. Cook 5 minutes. Return pork to the pot. Add the 1 ½ teaspoons of spice mixture. Add broth, hominy, and tomatoes. Bring to a boil. Reduce heat, cover halfway, and let simmer 25 minutes.

Tips

Use chicken instead of pork if you're trying to cut red meats. Keep this stew seasonal by changing out the veggies with whatever's in season.

51. Guinness Beef Stew

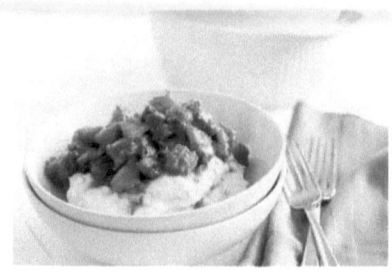

Summary

The addition of Guinness to this stew adds a whole new dimension of flavor that will keep you coming back for more.

Ingredients

- 2 lbs. Boneless Chuck Roast (cubed)
- 5 cups Onion (chopped)
- 4 cups Beef Broth
- 1 ¼ cup Whole Grain Flour
- 1 ½ cups Carrots (sliced)
- 1 ½ cup Parsnips (sliced)
- 1 cup Turnip (cubed)
- 1 (11.2 oz.) bottle Guinness Stout (or other stout beer)
- 3 Tbsps. Olive Oil
- 1 Tbsp. Tomato Paste
- 1 Tbsp. Raisins
- 2 Tbsps. Parsley
- 1 tsp Caraway Seeds
- 1 tsp Salt
- ½ tsp Black Pepper

Method

1. Heat oil in a large pan on medium-high heat. Add beef and cook until browned. Remove beef and set aside. Add onion. Cook 5 minutes. Stir

in tomato paste. Cook 1 minute. Stir in beer and broth. Add the beef back in.

2. Add salt, raisins, caraway seeds, and pepper. Bring to a boil. Reduce heat, cover and let simmer 1 hour. Stir occasionally. Remove lid, bring to a boil. Cook 50 minutes, stirring occasionally. Add carrot, turnip, and parsnip. Reduce heat to low and simmer for 30 minutes or until vegetables are tender.

Fun Facts

Here's 3 reasons you want to add more dark beer to your diet: Flavonoids found in dark beer help break up blood clots. Dark beer is also packed with iron. A bottle of dark beer a day can reduce your risk of kidney stones by up to 40%.

52. Make Ahead Beef Rolls

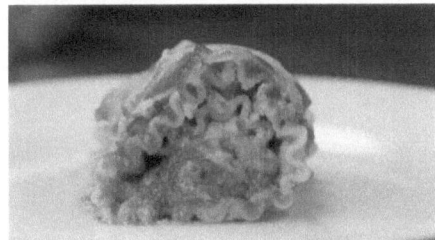

Summary

These surprisingly healthy morsels will please the whole family.

Ingredients

- 6 cups Whole Grain Flour
- 3 tsp Active Dry Yeast
- 4 ½ Tbsp. Butter
- 4 ½ tsp Honey
- 2 tsp Salt
- 2 Tbsp. Milk
- 2 cups Warm Water
- 1 ½ lbs. Ground Beef
- 1 medium head Cabbage (shredded)
- 1 lbs. Mozzarella (shredded)
- 1-3 Chiles (hot, diced)

- 2 cloves Garlic (minced)
- 1 large Onion (chopped)
- Olive Oil
- Salt & Pepper to Taste

Method

1. In a bowl, combine warm water and yeast. Let sit 5 minutes. Add butter, honey, salt, and milk. Mix well. Stir in flour 1 cup at a time. Mix until a ball forms. Turn out onto floured surface. Knead until smooth (about 5 minutes). Cover with a damp cloth and set somewhere warm until it doubles in size. Heat oil in a large pan on medium high heat. Add beef and cabbage. Cook until beef is browned. Add salt and pepper to taste.

2. Divide dough into roll-sized pieces. Flatten each roll and fill with a spoonful of beef mixture. Sprinkle cheese on top. Fold over and pinch the sides to seal. Brush the tops with oil. Bake for about 50 minutes at 350°F or until golden.

Tips

Try these alternatives to ground beef for an even healthier meal: Shredded chicken. Spinach and feta cheese. Homemade tuna salad.

53. Black Bean & Sweet Potato Empanadas

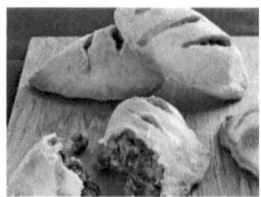

Summary

The combination of black beans and sweet potatoes makes for an irresistible lunch or dinner.

Ingredients

- 2 cups Whole Grain Flour
- ¼ cup Cold Water
- 1 large Egg (beaten)

- ¾ tsp Salt
- 1/3 cup Olive Oil
- 1 Tbsp. Cider Vinegar
- 1 Tbsp. Cumin
- 1 cup Mashed Sweet Potatoes
- 1 cup Black Beans
- 1/3 cup Green Onions (chopped)
- 1 Egg White (beaten)
- 2 Tbsps. Cilantro
- 1 tsp Chili Powder
- ½ tsp Salt

Method

1. In a large bowl, combine flour and ¾ teaspoon salt. In another bowl, blend ¼ cup water, egg, oil, and vinegar. Gradually add water mixture to flour. Mix until it forms a ball. Wrap dough in plastic wrap and let sit in the fridge 1 hour.

2. Toast cumin seeds in a pan over medium heat about 1 minute. In a bowl, add cumin seeds, sweet potatoes, ½ teaspoon salt, black beans, green onions, cilantro, chili powder, and egg white. Mix well. Dive dough into 10 balls. Roll each ball out into a circle (about 5" wide).

3. Divide the filling evenly onto each dough circle. Fold over and press the edges down with a fork. Place them on a greased baking sheet. Cut 3 slits across the top. Bake for about 15 minutes at 400°F or until lightly browned.

Fun Facts

Black beans help speed up digestion which helps you lose weight. The high fiber content works to sweep out toxins from your system. Their high phytonutrient content helps lower cholesterol.

54. Make Ahead Samosas

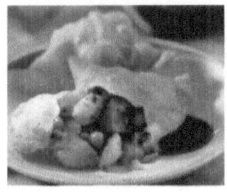

Summary

Dip these rich and hearty samosas in sour cream, sweet & source sauce, or a fresh mint chutney for a simple yet wholesome lunch or dinner.

Ingredients

- 8 sheets frozen Phyllo Dough (thawed)
- 1 cup Mashed Potatoes
- 2/3 cup Frozen Peas (thawed)
- 2/3 cup Carrot (shredded)
- ¼ cup Onion (chopped)
- 2 Tbsps. Olive Oil
- 2 tsp Mustard Seeds
- 1 ½ tsp Garam Masala
- ½ tsp Salt

Method

1. Heat oil in a pan on medium heat. Add onion. Cook 2 minutes. Add carrots. Cook 2 minutes. Add peas, mustard seeds, salt, and garam masala. Cook 2 minutes. Mix in potatoes. Remove from heat. Cut phyllo dough sheets into 3 strips (about 3"x14"). Spoon a portion of potato mixture onto the end of the strip. Fold that end over itself so that it forms a triangle shape at the tip.

2. Fold this triangle down. Continue to fold down until you reach the other end of the strip. Repeat for each samosa. Place samosas on a baking sheet. Brush with oil. Bake for about 20 minutes at 350° F or until lightly browned.

Tips

Make a large batch of phyllo dough from scratch to keep on hand for samosas and other yummy pastries. Use sweet potatoes, ginger, coconut milk, and cinnamon as filling for a sweet dessert. Get creative. You can stuff your samosa with just about anything.

5. Sweet Potato Burritos

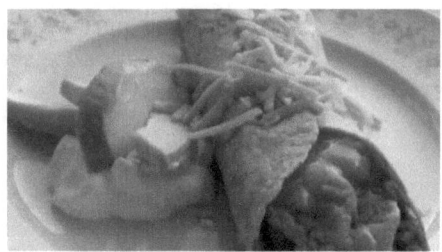

Summary

These irresistible burritos are perfect for a quick lunch or dinner.

Ingredients

- 6 cups Kidney Beans
- 4 cups Mashed Sweet Potatoes
- 2 cups Whole Grain Flour
- 1 cup Warm Water
- 3 Tbsps. Butter (melted)
- 1 tsp Salt
- ½ cup Cheddar (shredded)
- 1 large onion (chopped)
- 4 cloves Garlic (minced)
- 2 cups Water
- 3 Tbsps. Chili Powder
- 1 Tbsp. Olive Oil
- 4 tsp Mustard
- 2 tsp Cumin
- 3 Tbsps. Soy Sauce
- Cayenne Pepper to Taste

Method

1. In a large bowl, combine flour, warm water, and melted butter. Mix until it forms into a ball. Divide into approximately 24 small balls. Roll out each ball into a flat circle (about ¼" thick).

2. Cook each tortilla in a pan over medium-high heat until it bubbles up. Heat oil in a pan on medium-high heat. Add onions and garlic. Cook 3 minutes. Mash in the beans. Gradually stir in water. Remove from heat. Add soy sauce, cumin, mustard, chili powder, and cayenne pepper.

3. Divide the mashed bean mixture and mashed sweet potatoes evenly among the tortillas. Fold up the tortillas and place on a baking sheet. Bake for about 12 minutes at 350° F.

Fun Facts

Sweet potatoes are a fantastic source of most essential minerals. They help stabilize blood sugar levels which lowers the risk for diabetes and helps you lose weight. They also contain powerful cancer-fighting antioxidants.

56. Quick Wraps

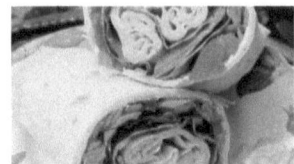

Summary

These wraps are easy to make and extremely satisfying—perfect to take to work.

Ingredients

- 2 cups Whole Grain Flour
- 1 cup Warm Water
- 2 Tbsps. Butter (melted)
- 2 cups Brown Rice
- 4 cups Water
- 4 (15 oz.) cans Black Beans
- 2 (15 oz.) cans Pinto Beans
- 1 (10 oz.) can Whole Kernel Corn
- 1 (10 oz.) can Diced Tomatoes and Green Chilies
- 2 cups Cheddar (shredded)

Method

1. Follow the first 4 steps in the previous recipe to make tortillas with the flour, warm water, and melted butter. Combine rice and water in a pot. Bring to a boil. Reduce to low heat, cover, and let simmer for about 20 minutes or until water is completely absorbed.

2. Transfer to a large bowl. Add beans, corn, tomatoes, chilies, and cheese. Mix well. Divide mixture evenly amongst the tortillas. Individually wrap each in plastic wrap. Heat in microwave for 2-3 minutes or until cooked through.

Tips

Try 2 or 3 different fillings to keep your lunches interesting. Swap corn for hominy to up the nutrition value. Swap quinoa for corn for even more whole grain benefits.

57. Cheesy Chive Loaf

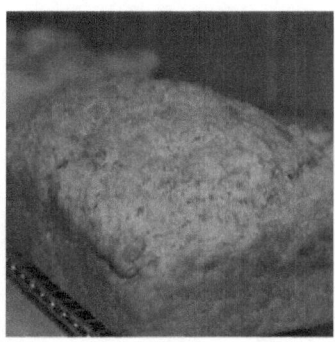

Summary

This is the perfect bread to eat along with any of the soups in this book.

Ingredients

- 5 ¼ cup Whole Grain Flour
- 1 cup Warm Milk (about 100° to 110° F)
- 1 package Active Dry Yeast (about 2 ¼ tsp)
- 5 large Egg Yolks
- 4 large Eggs (whole, divided)
- ¾ cup Fontina Cheese (shredded)
- 1 tsp Sugar
- 3 Tbsps. Butter (melted, plus more for greasing)
- 1 ½ tsp Salt
- ½ cup Chives (chopped)
- 2 Tbsps. Water
- 2 Tbsps. Parmesan (grated)

Method

1. Combine yeast and warm milk in a large bowl. Let sit 5 minutes. Blend in butter, salt, and egg yolks. Stir in cheese and chives. Stir in flour 1 cup at a time until it forms into a ball.

2. Turn dough out on a floured surface. Knead until smooth (but still slightly sticky). Cover in a damp towel and let rise in a warm place until doubled in size. Beat 1 egg and 2 tablespoons water until foamy. Brush the top of the loaf with the mixture. Sprinkle with parmesan. Bake for 25 minutes at 375° F or until golden.

Fun Facts

Whole grains not only contain a high dosage of fiber but also a surprising amount of protein. Whole grains stabilize blood sugar levels protecting you from diabetes and other diet-related problems.

58. Buttermilk Whole Grain Pancakes

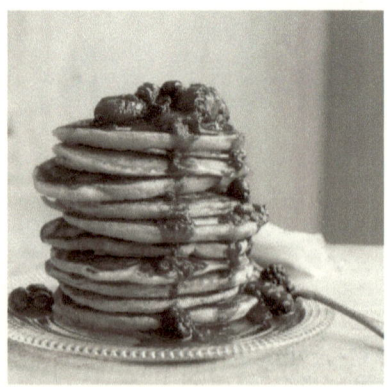

Summary

The whole grain provides fiber and flavor, making a hearty yet light and fluffy pancake.

Ingredients

- 1 ½ cups Whole Grain Flour
- 1 ½ cups Buttermilk
- 2 Tbsps. Butter (melted)
- 2 large Eggs

- 3 tsp Baking Powder
- 1 tsp Baking Soda
- 1 tsp Salt
- 1-3 Tbsps. Butter

Method

1. In a large bowl, combine flour, baking powder, baking soda, and salt. Add buttermilk, eggs, and melted butter. Mix until bubbly and free of clumps. Heat 1 tablespoon butter in a pan over medium-high heat. Ladle out pancake batter into pan.

2. Cook until the top begins to bubble then flip and cook the other side for 1-2 minutes or until cooked through. Repeat until the batter is gone. You may need to add another tablespoon of butter after every few pancakes.

Tips

Try adding any of the following ingredients right into the batter:

- *1 Banana (mashed, and an extra banana sliced for a topping)*
- *½ cup Fresh Blueberries*
- *½ cup Dark Chocolate (at least 70% cocoa, chopped)*

59. Cherry Chocolate Cookies

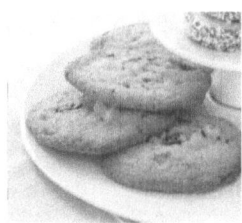

Summary

Enjoy these scrumptious treats guilt-free because they are actually highly nutritious.

Ingredients

- 2/3 Cup Whole Grain Flour
- 1 ½ Cups Rolled Oats

- 1 tsp Baking Soda
- ½ tsp Salt
- 6 Tbsps. Butter (plus extra for greasing)
- ¾ Cup Brown Sugar
- 1 Cup Dried Cherries
- 1 large Egg (beaten)
- 3 oz. dark chocolate, coarsely chopped

Method

1. In a large bowl, combine flour, baking soda, salt, and oats. In a small pan, melt butter. Remove from heat, add sugar. Add butter mixture and egg to flour mixture. Mix thoroughly. Add cherries and dark chocolate. Mix well.

2. Divide dough into 2"-3" balls. Lightly grease a baking sheet with butter or olive oil. Press the balls onto baking sheet. Bake for 12 minutes at 350° F.

Fun Facts

The copper in cherries helps keep skin young and healthy. Cherries are high in vitamin C which helps your immune system. Studies have found that cherries help get rid of belly flab.

60. Lamb Tagine

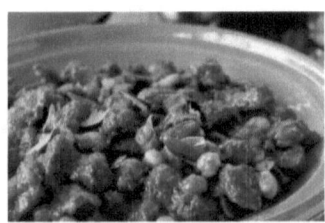

Summary

The carrot and the butternut present in this dish is a real winner with the kinds as well as with the mums, because they are so healthy!

Ingredients

- Olive oil
- 2 small onion, finely diced

- 1 carrot, finely diced (about 150g)
- 1kg lamb
- 2 fat cloves garlic, crushed
- ½ tsp. ground ginger, saffron, cumin, cinnamon powder
- 2 tbsp. clear honey
- 1 stock cube
- Butternut squash, peeled, cut into 1cm
- Handful of dried apricots, quartered
- Couscous

Method

1. Heat olive oil; add carrots and onions and cook till softened. Follow with the chopped lamb, garlic and spices. Sauté till aromatic.

2. Now honey, apricots, stock cube and water and cover to cook the meat on simmer for about an hour. Add the squash in and cook for about half an hour more until lamb and squash are tender. Serve with couscous.

Fun Facts

The tagine is a one-pot, slow cooked dish which is easy to prepare and will satisfy the entire family.

61. Crispy Bacon with Cauliflower Pasta

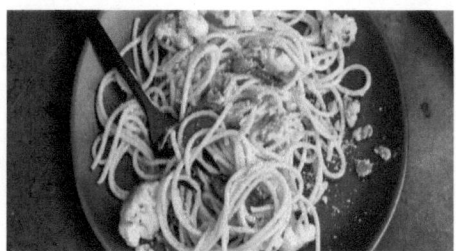

Summary

It cannot get better than healthy cauliflower and tasty bacon in one family friendly bake is great, eaten with a side of garlic bread.

Ingredients

- 2 small cauliflower, cut into florets

- Streaky bacon
- 1 packet pasta
- Butter
- Milk
- Plain flour
- 150g grated cheddar
- 2 tsp. Dijon mustard
- ½ cup breadcrumbs

Method

1. Fry bacon slices and keep aside. Bring a large pot of water with salt to the boil to cook the pasta. In the last 10 minutes, add florets to the water too. Meanwhile, in a separate pan, make a simple roux with seasoning, mustard and cheese.

2. Put florets, pasta and reserved pasta water into pan with cheese sauce and bacon. Sprinkle breadcrumbs and the remaining cheese and grill for until browned.

Fun Facts

Did you know that cauliflower is an excellent source of Vitamin C that helps in keeping you super healthy?

62. Fishy Fish Pie

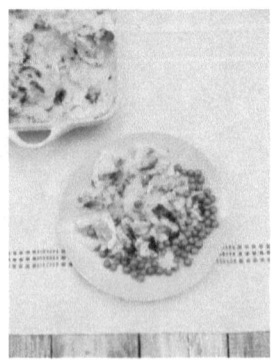

Summary

Simple and very easy to prepare, this dish can even be portioned into small bowls for easy service for the kids!

Ingredients

- 1.5kg potatoes, peeled and halved
- Some butter, milk and flour
- 3 spring onions, finely sliced
- 1 packet fish pie mix
- Splash of Dijon or English mustard
- Handful of small bunch chives, finely snipped
- 1 handful frozen sweet corn
- Grated cheddar

Method

1. Add potatoes to saucepan with enough water and simmer until cooked through. Once done, drain and mash them with seasoning and butter. Take another pan and add butter, flour and onions and sauté. Slowly pour in the milk and whisk continuously, bringing it to a slow boil.

2. Once it thickens, take it off the heat and add the cheese, mustard, fish, chives and corn. Spoon the above mixture into an oven dish. Add the potato mixture on top and sprinkle with cheese and breadcrumbs, and bake for about half an hour.

Fun Facts

Fish such as salmon and tuna are rich in Omega-3 fatty acids which are the kind of fats that are good for health.

63. Eggplant and Sausages

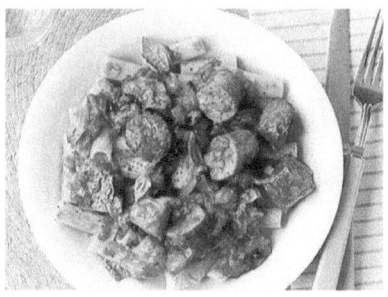

Summary

Juicy pork sausages combined with the goodness of ratatouille and courgettes!

Ingredients

- 1 onion, cut into 16 wedges
- 3 courgettes, cut into bite-sized pieces
- 1 red pepper, cut into bite-sized pieces
- Olive oil
- 8 pork sausages
- 3 garlic cloves, crushed
- 400g can chopped tomatoes

Method

1. Cook the cut onions, red peppers and courgettes in an oiled baking dish for about 20 minutes in a 220-degree heated oven. Fry the sausages on a pan, side by side, until browned. Remove baking dish and add in garlic and tomatoes. Top it up with the sausages and cook again for about 15 minutes until veggies are tender.

Fun Facts

Zucchini is a great source of Vitamin C as well as Vitamin A.

64. Chili Pasta with Cauliflowers

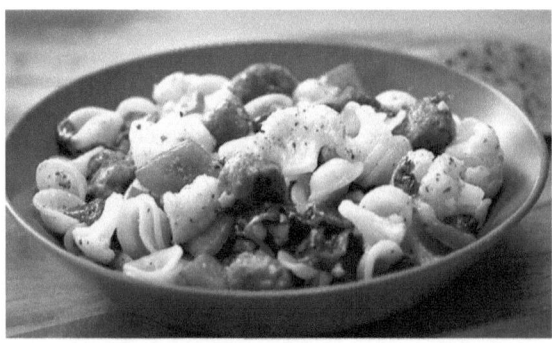

Summary

Pasta is always a wholesome dish for any family and healthy as well.

Ingredients

- 2 cauliflowers, chopped into small florets
- 6 strips streaky bacon, cut into large pieces

- ½ tsp. chili powder
- 500g pasta of your choice
- 200g tub cherry tomatoes
- Handful basil leaves, roughly torn

Method

1. First steam cauliflower for 5 minutes while you shallow fry the bacon with chili powder. Then add in the cauliflower florets and cook in the same bacon fat.

2. Follow it up with the tomatoes once cauliflower is cooked. Meanwhile, cook pasta according to package instructions. Drain and add it to the bacon, tomato and cauliflower mixture. Serve with a scattering of basil leaves.

Fun Facts

Did you know that cauliflower remains white only due to the protective covering of the leaves around it, keeping away the sun?!

65. Different Mac n Cheese

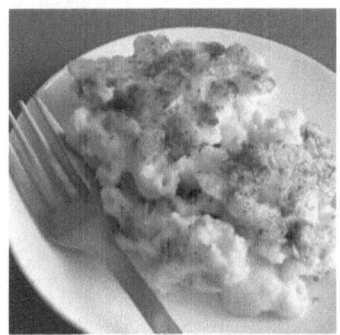

Summary

Comforting and creamy, this bake will make sure that the entire family is waiting at the table for dinner!

Ingredients

- 2 small butternut squash, cut in chunks
- 3 tsp. olive oil

- 1 packet macaroni
- 100g butter
- 75g plain flour
- Pinch of English mustard powder
- Half litre milk
- 250g cheddar cheese, grated
- 75gg parmesan, grated

Method

1. Add squash with olive oil plus salt into a baking dish and add to the oven for about 20 minutes, while you cook the macaroni side by side. In a skillet, add butter, mustard powder and flour and whisk. Then slowly pour the milk to make a smooth paste.

2. Remove sauce from the heat, add in cheddar and a little bit of squash and mash it all in. Season and then add in the macaroni along with leftover squash and pour into the oven proof dish. Bake for 20 minutes until browned.

Fun Facts

Butternut is a type of squash and contains the highest levels of Vitamin A and carotenes.

66. Easy Cheese Pizza

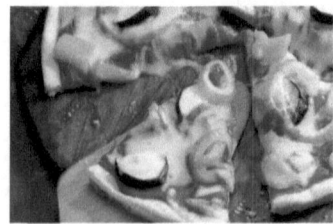

Summary

Who doesn't love a cheese pizza and when it is so easy to make, children and parents are equally happy!

Ingredients

- Ready thin bases

For the sauce

- 150ml tomato sauce
- Handful fresh basil
- 2 garlic cloves, crushed

For the topping

- 150g sliced mozzarella
- Shaved parmesan
- Cherry tomatoes, cut in half

Method

1. For the sauce, mix basil, crushed garlic and tomato together along with seasoning. Add water if you want to thin it down just a tad bit. Smoothen the sauces over the base and add in the cheese and tomatoes over it. Drizzle a little bit of olive oil and seasoning. Bake for about ten minutes or until crisp and cheese melted. Pizza is ready to serve with a garnish of fresh basil leaves.

Fun Facts

Cheese contains phosphorous, zinc, calcium and protein all together. Since it is a milk product it is known to be healthy is adequate limits.

67. Easy Tomato Soup

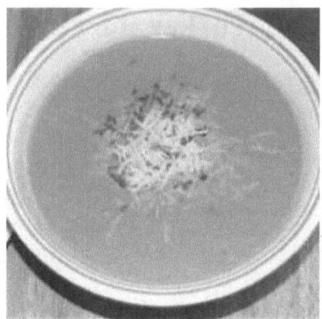

Summary

Tomatoes are filled with nutrients and anti-oxidants that help in building immunity for the body. It is also a wholesome meal for the family and kids.

Ingredients

- 400g can cherry tomatoes
- 1 tbsp caster sugar
- 100ml vegetable stock
- Dash each Tabasco and Worcestershire sauce
- 2 tbsp mascarpone
- few torn basil leaves (optional)

For the dipping items

- 1 medium ciabatta roll, halved
- 1 garlic clove, halved
- 125g ball mozzarella cheese, shredded

Method

1. Add tomatoes, stock, sugar and sauces into a pan with seasoning and bring to a slow simmer. Remove off the heat and stir in the mascarpone and whisk till it blends. For the dippers: heat grill and toast the ciabata. Rub some garlic and salt on it and top with cheese and grill. Slice it up into thin finger like slices and serve.

Fun Facts

Tomatoes are rich in anti-oxidants. It is interesting to know that they also fight cancer and also improves vision.

68. Turkey Burgers

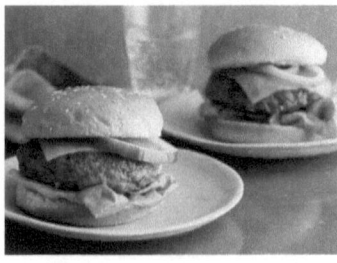

Summary

Shape turkey thigh mince into these easy patties and serve between burger bread for a great dinner!

Ingredients

- pound turkey thigh mince
- 1kg sweet potatoes, peeled and cut into chips
- 1 packet cheddar, grated
- 4 tbsp. olive oil
- 1 small cucumber, sliced thin
- 3 spring onions, finely chopped
- 4 burger patties
- Splash of tomato ketchup

Method

1. Add turkey mince to a bowl with cheddar, spring onions and seasoning and mix. Then shape these into patties for 4 burgers. Put in the chips of sweet potato in a baking tray with a drizzle of olive oil and salt. Cook for about half an hour.

2. Cook the burger breads for about 10 minutes on both sides and add the burger patty on one side. Top with cucumber and ketchup and cover with the other bread. Serve with a side of hot sweet potato chips.

Fun Facts

Did you know that sweet potatoes are believed to be healthier than normal potatoes? They are also tastier!

69. Chicken Curry with Sweet Potatoes

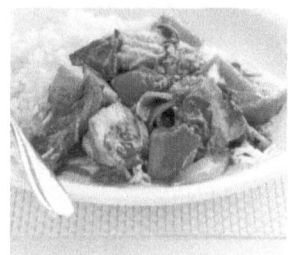

Summary

If you like a little Indian spice in your dishes, then this curry is perfect to host another family over for curry dinners!

Ingredients

- 1 tbsp. sunflower oil
- 1 onion, chopped
- 450g boneless, skinless chicken thighs, cut into pieces
- 1 jar Korma paste
- 2 garlic cloves, crushed
- 500g sweet potatoes, cut into small chunks
- 400g can chopped tomatoes
- 100g baby spinach
- Basmati rice, to serve

Method

1. First sauté the onions and then add the chicken pieces and brown. Add curry paste, garlic and then water, tomatoes and sweet potatoes. Simmer till chicken and sweet potato is cooked. Check for seasoning and add the spinach till it wilts. Serve with basmati.

Fun Facts

Great Indian styled curry to add to your list of good recipes.

70. Ratatouille Salad

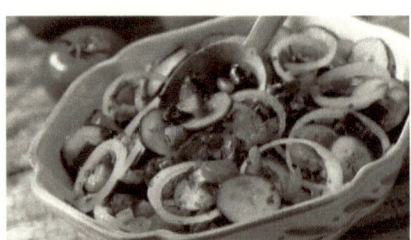

Summary

This rustic vegetable is seen in French origins and mixes well with the Mediterranean cuisine.

Ingredients

- 2 large aubergines, sliced lengthwise
- 4 small courgettes, sliced lengthwise
- 2 red or yellow peppers, sliced lengthwise

- 4 large ripe tomatoes, cut lengthwise
- 5 tbsp. olive oil
- Supermarket pack or small bunch basil
- 1 medium onion, peeled and thinly sliced
- 3 garlic cloves, peeled and crushed
- 1 tbsp. red wine vinegar
- 1 tsp. sugar (any kind)

Method

1. Cut all of the vegetables lengthwise and add to a large bowl. Heat a skillet and add aborigines to it and fry followed by courgettes and peppers. Then add onions and garlic and add all the sautéed vegetables to the bowl.

2. Add vinegar, sugar and tomatoes and half the quantity of basil. Add seasoning and mix it all up. Garnish with remaining basil and serve.

Fun Facts

You can even add in a splash of harissa paste along with chickpeas and olives, to give the dish a more Mediterranean feel.

71. Bean and Sausages in a Pot

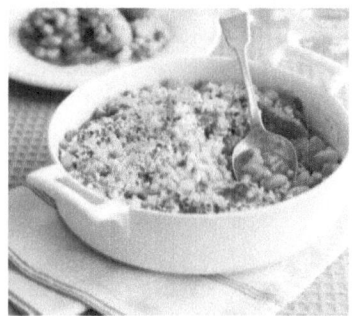

Summary

The goodness of sausage mixed with the healthiness of beans all in one pot!

Ingredients

- 10 large sausages
- 1 tsp. mustard sauce

- ½ can tomato sauce
- 1 tbsp. brown sugar
- 3 cans butter beans

Method

1. Start by frying off sausages until they are browned. Add tomato sauce with sugar and then add the beans, and mustard. Bring this mixture to simmer for about 30 minutes. Serve with herbed rice.

Fun Facts

This super-fast recipe is wholesome and very easy to make. You can even add all of this to the oven and bake till browned.

72. Chili Cheese Mac n Cheese

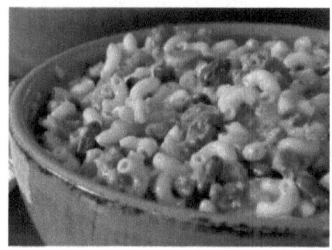

Summary

For those who don't like the cheesy macaroni, here's a slightly spicier version of the same.

Ingredients

- 1 teaspoon garlic powder
- 1 teaspoon olive oil
- ¾ pound ground round
- 1 teaspoon ground cumin
- 1 teaspoon ground coriander
- 2 cups fat-free, lower-sodium beef broth
- 2 teaspoons chilli powder
- 1 cup water
- 1 can mild diced tomatoes and green chills, untrained
- 8 ounces uncooked elbow macaroni
- 1/2 cup fat-free milk

- 4 ounces 1/3-less-fat cream cheese
- 4 1/2 ounces finely shredded reduced-fat sharp cheddar cheese

Method

1. Heat a pan. Add oil, beef and all the ground powders plus garlic and sauté. Add the stock, tomatoes and water and bring to a simmer. Add in the macaroni and cover and cook.

2. In another pan stir in milk and cream cheese over medium heat until cheese melts. Stir in the cheddar cheese and then add this sauce to the macaroni pot and toss.

Fun Facts

This recipe is not only a different change for the kids but also for the parents!

73. Pita Pockets

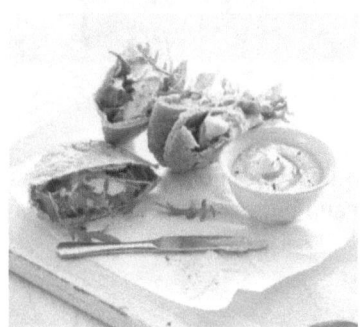

Summary

This protein rich dish is a great option when you are having extended family over for dinner. It is easy, filling and overall, a healthy meal option.

Ingredients

- 1 whole wheat pita pocket
- ¼ cup of hummus mixed with any leftover grains or beans.
- ½ sliced avocado
- Slices of iceberg lettuce
- Roasted slices of pepper
- Salt and pepper to taste

Method

1. Mix beans, hummus and grains with seasoning in a bowl. Line pita pockets with hummus on both sides. Add slices of avocado and red pepper. You can even grill it before serving.

Fun Facts

This recipe tastes best when grilled and served warm.

74. Pesto Sandwiches

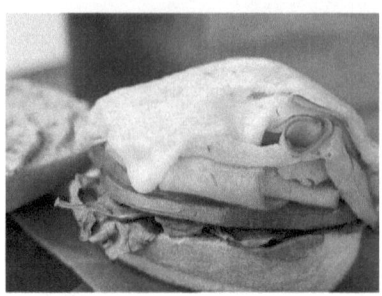

Summary

Sandwiches are the yummiest and most filling options for breakfast. Fill it up with any item you desire and butter it, and they will have to taste good!

Ingredients

- 1 can pesto sauce, store bought or home made
- 1 zucchini, sliced
- 1 onion, sliced
- 1 packet of brown bread
- Butter
- 6-8 button mushrooms, sliced
- 1 small broccoli, cut into small florets
- Handful of olives

Method

1. First butter bread slices and then line with pesto sauce. Add sliced vegetables thereafter and sprinkle olives on top. Cover with the top slice of bread and place on the grill, buttering both sides. Serve hot!

Fun Facts

Sandwiches are one of the fastest selling options for a quick bite. It is wholesome and healthy.

75. Baked Dish with Veggies

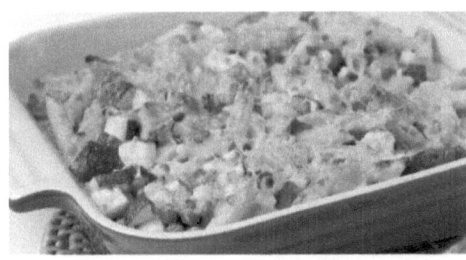

Summary

Perfect for a Sunday night meal to end your weekend with, before you start off on a hectic week! Also makes for super snacking option in between meals.

Ingredients

- 2-3 tbsp. olive oil
- 2 cups chopped onion
- 3-4 garlic cloves, minced
- ½ pound soya chunks, crumbled
- 1 ½ cup diced bell peppers
- 6 cups white or brown bread, cubed
- 1 tbsp. Dijon mustard
- 12 eggs
- 1 ½ cups grated cheese
- 2 cups milk
- Salt and pepper, to taste

Method

1. Heat a skillet and add garlic, onions and bell peppers in the same order. Layer bread pieces in a single line on a lined baking tray and follow with soya chunks. Brush with mustard and sprinkle a good layer of cheese above. In a separate bowl, whisk salt, pepper, milk and cheese and eggs well and pour over the soya chunks layer and bake for about an hour in a preheated oven.

Fun Facts

While this is a pure vegetarian recipe, the soya chunks can be replaced for chicken pieces as well!

76. Shrimp and Spinach Pasta

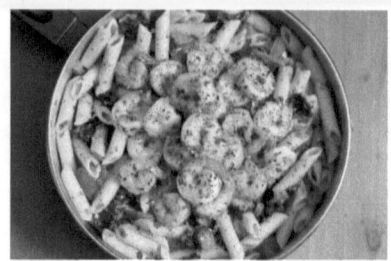

Summary

The shrimp and spinach lend a wonderful flavor to the entire pasta dish!

Ingredients

- 1 packet fusilli, or other short pasta
- 3 tablespoons unsalted butter
- Salt and black pepper
- 1kg medium shrimp (raw)
- 1 large leek, chopped
- 1 cup heavy cream
- 12 cups baby spinach
- Zest of 1 lemon

Method

1. Cook pasta and reserve a little of the water. In another skillet, add butter, leeks, salt, and pepper and cover till leeks soften. Now add shrimp and zest of lemon followed by the rest of the ingredients. Add cream and salt to pasta pot and then add the shrimp mix and toss to coat.

Fun Facts

The shrimp in this recipe is lightly cooked and thus providing a lot of nutrients to the dish.

77. Shrimp and Olive Salad

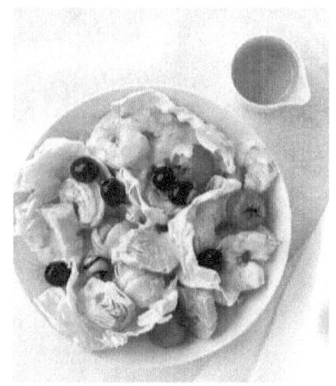

Summary

This Mediterranean inspired shrimp salad with couscous is definitely a onetime meal, making everyone beg for repeats!

Ingredients

- 1 10-ounce box couscous (1 1/3 cups)
- 1 tablespoon olive oil
- 1 small onion, chopped
- 1 28-ounce can diced tomatoes, drained
- 3/4 cup pitted green olives
- 1/2 cup dry white wine (such as Sauvignon Blanc)
- Kosher salt and pepper
- pound medium shrimp, peeled and deveined

Method

1. First cook couscous according to instructions. In another saucepan, add oil, onion and sauté. Follow with tomatoes, olives and wine and seasoning. Simmer and stir till it thickens. Serve with the couscous.

Fun Facts

Couscous is a wholesome Mediterranean meal that is one of their main meals. Just like other regions survive on bread or rice as a wholesome constant, couscous represents the same.

78. Asian Salmon with Bok Choy

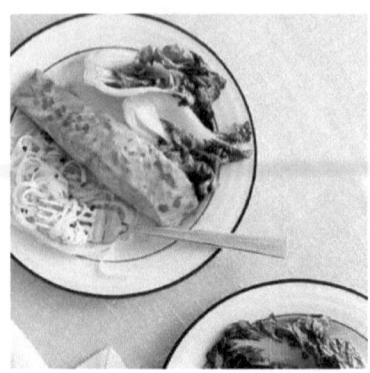

Summary

Salmon is a fish that is rich in Omega-3 fatty acids which is extremely healthy and good for health.

Ingredients

- 1 cup long-grain white rice
- 2 tablespoons honey
- 1 tablespoon soy sauce
- 1/4 teaspoon crushed red pepper
- 4 6-ounce skinless salmon fillets
- pound baby bok choy

Method

1. Cook rice according to packet instructions. In another bowl, mix honey, soy sauce and red peppers. Next step is to broil salmon fillets basted with the honey mix. On the side, steam the baby Bok Choy and serve with the salmon and a side portion of rice.

Fun Facts

Depending on how you like your vegetables, you can steam it for a longer or shorter portion of time.

79. Salmon and Fennel Salad

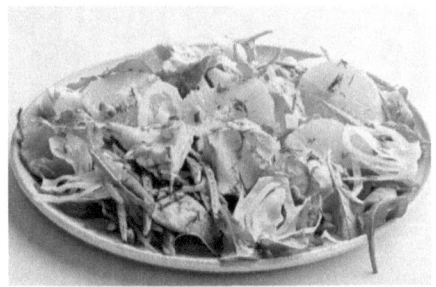

Summary

The fennel provides a good contrast to the otherwise smelly fish!

Ingredients

- 4 salmon fillets
- 2 tablespoon olive oil
- Salt and black pepper
- 3/4 cup plain low-fat Greek yogurt
- A lemon, thinly sliced
- 1 fennel, cored and thinly sliced
- 1 small cucumber, thinly sliced
- 2 tsp. cider vinegar
- Rye bread, for serving

Method

1. Rub salmon with oil and place on a baking dish with a sprinkle of cayenne pepper and salt. Put in lemon slices on top and bake till just cooked through. Take another bowl and add vinegar, yoghurt, salt and pepper. Add the fennels, cucumbers and gently stir together. Serve salmon with a side of the salad!

Fun Facts

Fennel is said to be a great mouth freshener, making this a perfect accompaniment to a fish meal!

80. Chicken with Prosciutto

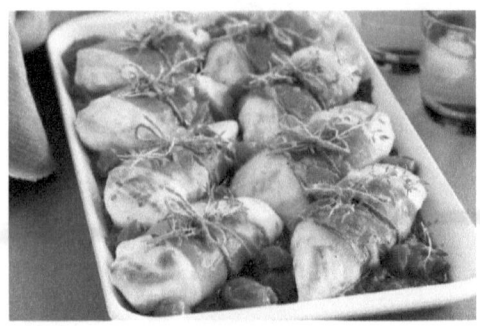

Summary

The best of two meats, combined in one dish!

Ingredients

- 4 boneless, skinless chicken breasts
- 8-10 slices prosciutto
- 2 small zucchini, thinly sliced into half-moons
- 2 tablespoons olive oil
- 2 clove garlic, thinly sliced
- 1/2 teaspoon salt and pepper
- 1 lemon

Method

1. Season chicken with salt and pepper and place in skillet and cook for about 2 minutes on each side. In another skillet, cook prosciutto till crispy. Follow with zucchini, garlic and salt and pepper and cook. Now add the above mixture to the chicken pan. Squeeze lime from top and mix gently. Serve in plates.

Fun Facts

Include a few tips here about the dish, or include a few fun facts about some of the ingredients. For example, if the main ingredient in this recipe was broccoli, write the title "3 Reasons Broccoli Helps Reduce Cholesterol", and then just write down the 3 reasons.

81. Turkey and Broccoli Pasta

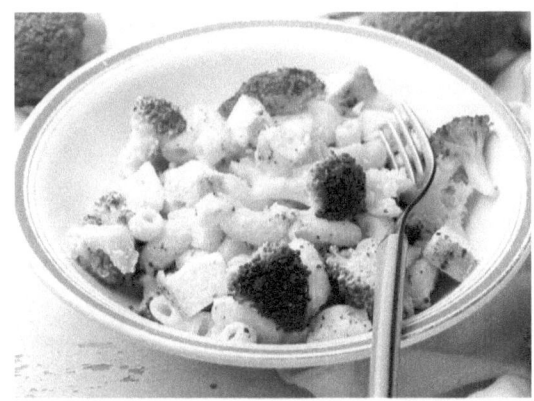

Summary

Broccoli may not exactly be your child's favorite vegetable but that can be compensated with the turkey! It's pasta after all, they won't be able to resist it!

Ingredients

- 3/4-pound orecchiette or any pasta shape
- 3 tablespoons olive oil
- 2 cups broccoli florets
- 2 cloves garlic, chopped
- pound ground turkey
- 1/2 teaspoon crushed red pepper
- 1 teaspoon fennel seed
- Kosher salt
- Parmesan, for serving

Method

1. Cook pasta as mentioned on the packet. Add broccoli in the end and drain water out immediately. In a skillet, add oil, turkey, garlic, fennel seeds and rec pepper and cook till meat is browned. Season with salt. Gently mix pasta and broccoli with oil and serve with sprinkle of cheese.

Fun Facts

Turkey is a rich source of protein, and skinless turkey is also low in fat.

82. Beef Chili

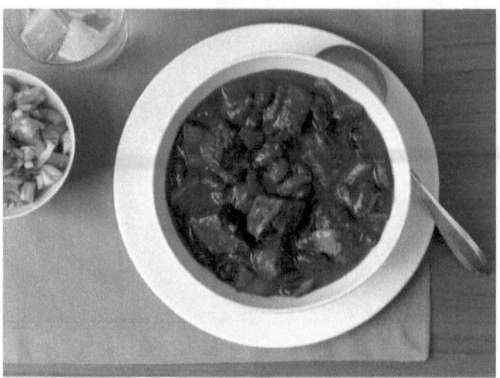

Summary

Who doesn't love a good portion of beef? Your kids will definitely enjoy this one!

Ingredients

- Olive oil
- 3 carrots, chopped
- 2 onions, chopped
- 1-pound ground beef
- 2 bell peppers, chopped
- 3 tablespoons tomato paste
- 2 tablespoon chili powder
- 2 15-ounce cans black beans, rinsed
- 1 cup corn kernels (from 1 ear, or frozen and thawed)
- Salt and black pepper
- 1/2 cup grated Cheddar (2 ounces)
- 3 spring onions, sliced

Method

1. Sauté onions, carrots and peppers in a skillet with oil. Add beef and cook till pinkish brown. Follow with tomato paste and cook. Add beans, water, chili powder, salt and pepper. Simmer and then add the corn kernels. Split it between bowls and top with grated cheese and spring onions.

Fun Facts

One of the tastiest meats known to man is beef! While it is a fatty meat, it also has a hell of a lot of proteins filled in it.

83. Kale and Tomato Spaghetti

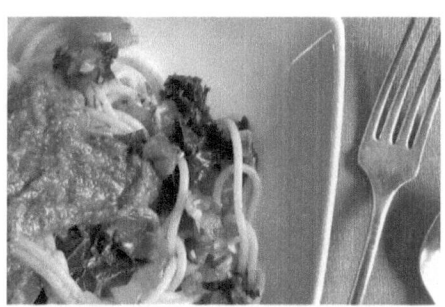

Summary

With ingredients such as kale and tomatoes, this recipe is a little less than super healthy!

Ingredients

- 1 packet spaghetti
- 2 small red onion, thinly sliced
- 3 tablespoons olive oil
- 2 small bunch kale, torn roughly
- 3 cloves garlic, chopped
- Salt and black pepper
- 1/4 cup chopped roasted almonds
- 1.5 pints grape tomatoes, halved
- 1/4 cup grated pecorino, plus more for serving

Method

1. Cook pasta according to instructions on the packet, reserving some pasta water. Heat a skillet, and garlic, onions salt and pepper and sauté. Add kale leaves and tomatoes and cook till they soften. In a separate bowl, add pasta, kale mixture, almonds, cheese and pasta cooking water and toss.

Fun Facts

2 reasons why kale is so good: 1 cup has only 33 calories and it's filled with Vitamin C, A and K!

84. Poached Fish

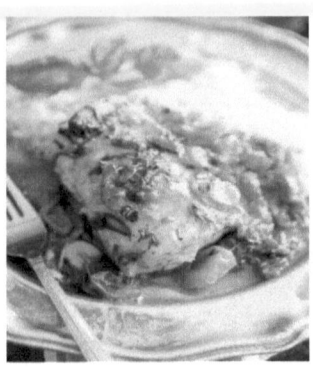

Summary

Do not fear if this recipe is served to kids, because the white wine used in the dish is evaporated by the end of the meal, and is added only for a slight flavor.

Ingredients

- Kosher salt and black pepper
- pound red potatoes
- 4 tablespoons unsalted butter
- ½ kilo green beans, trimmed
- 4 filleted fish, 6-ounce pieces each
- 2 tablespoons chopped fresh chives
- 3 cups white wine, for cooking

Method

1. First boil potatoes with salt. Add green beans to it in the end just for 5 minutes and then drain both. Heat a skillet with butter. Add salt, pepper, chives and mix.

2. Bring another skillet to heat. Add in the wine with the heat turned on high, and when just the quantity is slightly reduced, place the seasoned fish fillets into it and cover and cook for 4-5 minutes. Once

done, serve a slice each with a side of quartered potatoes, beans and chive butter.

Fun Facts

Poached fish is a healthy and different option of eating fish. Try poaching as opposed to baking or frying.

85. Green Grape Curry

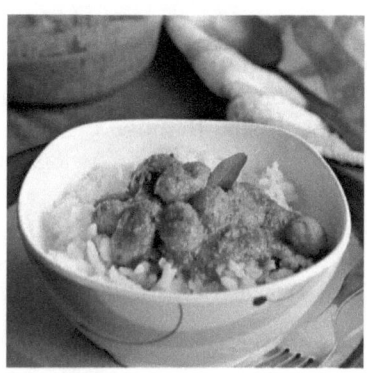

Summary

If your children love grapes, then here is the dish to make for them! Add it to an Indian styled curry and serve with bread!

Ingredients

- 2 onions, peeled and roughly chopped
- inch Ginger, peeled
- 10-12 small garlic cloves, peeled
- 2-3 green chili, depending on level of spiciness
- 100g cashew nuts
- 1 bay leaf
- Oil
- 50g melon seeds
- ¼ tsp. Red chili powder
- ¼ tsp. Turmeric powder
- Salt, to taste
- 1 tsp. Dry fenugreek leaves
- Garam masala, optional
- 200g-250g green grapes

- 1 tsp. chopped coriander
- 3 tbsp. fresh cream

Method

1. Add onion, garlic, ginger, melon seeds, green chilies and cashews to a pan with 1 cup water and bring to slow boil. Once done, turn off, let cool and then puree in a food processor. Heat oil in another skillet, add bay leaves, chili powder, turmeric powder, and onion paste. Let t cook.

2. Add a cup of water and bring to simmer. Follow with salt, kasooori methi (leaving some for garnish) and garam masala, if using. Pour in grapes and give gentle stir. Remove off heat and add cream. Serve with garnish of coriander leaves and few kasoori methi.

Fun Facts

Dried fenugreek leaves are extremely flavorful, and give out a very pleasing aroma to food.

86. Spanish Omelets

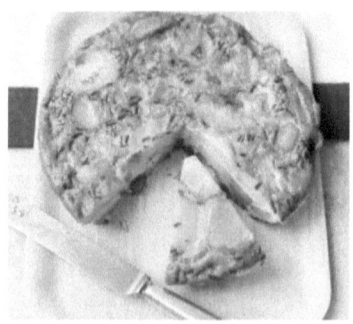

Summary

Who says you can't have an omelet for a meal? Serve this up as slightly late dinner with slices of buttered bread and enjoy!

Ingredients

- Olive oil
- 2 small onion, chopped
- 2.5 ounces Spanish chorizo, sliced thin

- pound potatoes, diced
- 3/4 cup flat-leaf parsley, roughly chopped
- Kosher salt and pepper
- 1 small green-leaf lettuce
- 1 cup, shredded Cheddar
- 10-12 large eggs, beaten
- 1/2 small red onion, thinly sliced

Method

1. Add onion to a hot skillet and sauté. Follow with salt and pepper, chorizo and potatoes and cover and cook. Add in a sprinkle of parsley. Pour eggs from a slight height and let it form an omelet. Sprinkle cheese on top and cover and cook on a low flame. Sprinkle with cheese and serve.

Fun Facts

You can even add all the above ingredients to a baking dish and bake it in the oven!

87. Baked Cod

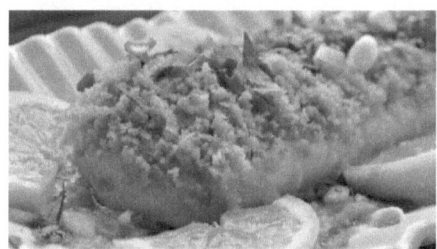

Summary

When a fish is baked, it retains more nutrients that when it is fried, and is also tastier most times.

Ingredients

- 4 pieces skinless fish filled of cod or sea bass fillet, 6-ounce each
- 4 tablespoons olive oil
- 12 small red potatoes, sliced 1/4 inch thick
- 1/2 teaspoon chili powder
- Salt and black pepper

- 1 lemon
- 3 bunches scallions, trimmed

Method

1. Bake potatoes with olive oil, chili powder, salt and pepper in the oven. Toss occasionally. Put fish and scallions on a hot skillet and cook for 2 minutes on each side. Place on a baking dish. Slice lemon thinly over the fish along with lime zest. Add the cooked potato and let the fish roast in the oven. Serve with lemon juice, optional.

Fun Facts

Just like salmon or tuna, cod is also a healthy fish containing Omega 3 fatty acids.

88. Sausage Stir-Fry

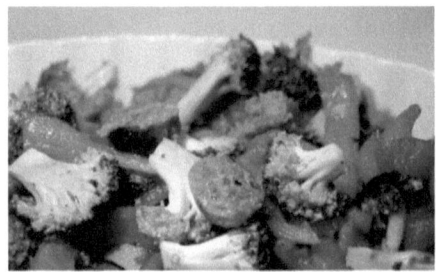

Summary

One of the fastest ways to cook sausage, and oh-so-yummy!

Ingredients

- 1 cup good quality sausages, chopped into 1 cm. chunks
- 1 red onion, finely chopped
- 3-4 garlic cloves, finely chopped
- 1 cup ketchup
- Salt and pepper, to taste
- ½ cup tomato puree
- 1 tsp. Worcestershire sauce
- Hot sauce or Tabasco sauce, as desired
- Water if needed

Method

1. Heat a skillet with oil and add onion and garlic and sauté. Follow it up with the sausages and cook till they brown. Then add in the ketchup, tad bit of tomato puree, salt and pepper and a pinch of Tabasco or any hot sauce and Worcestershire sauce. Cover and cook for two minutes.

Fun Facts

This sweet-spicy recipe allows you the best of both worlds with sausages. There are at least 30 different ways in which sausages can be used in recipes!

89. Chicken Mince Cutlets

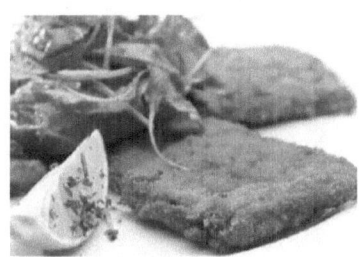

Summary

Cutlets are the easiest snack and meal recipes that are famous with kids of all ages. They are little powerhouses of food that are easy to handle.

Ingredients

- 400g chicken mince
- 2 red onions, finely chopped
- Oil, for cooking
- 1 tbsp. ginger garlic paste
- Salt and pepper
- ½ cup coriander leaves, chopped fine
- 1 tsp. chili powder
- ¼ tsp. turmeric powder
- ½ tsp. cumin powder
- ½ tsp. coriander powder
- day old potato mash
- 1-2 Egg beaten well
- Handful of bread crumbs

Method

1. Heat a skillet and add ginger garlic paste and onions and sauté. Add in the mince and break with the spoon. Follow this with the powders, seasoning and coriander leaves. Once free of all the water released, let the mixture cool and then add enough potato mash to hold the mixture. Then shape these into cutlets. While preparing cutlets, dip them into the beaten egg first, and then cover it with breadcrumbs by rolling it in and shallow fry.

Fun Facts

One of the easiest cutlet recipes which stores well even in the freezer and can be pulled out for a snack at any time!

90. Chickpea Salad

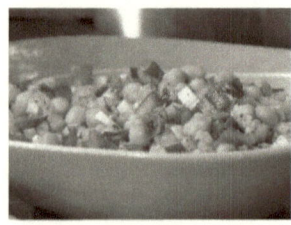

Summary

This Mediterranean inspired salad is a fresh burst of flavor in the mouth and is a healthy meal option for kids too.

Ingredients

- 1 can cooked chickpeas
- 1 red onion, finely chopped
- 1 tomato, finely chopped
- Handful of kalamata olives
- 1-2 tbsp. extra virgin olive oil
- 2 tbsp. hummus
- Pinch of sumac
- Pinch of harissa, if needed
- Salt and pepper
- 1 lemon, squeezed
- Fresh mint, for garnish

Method

1. Add the onions, tomato, olives and chickpeas to a bowl along with seasoning and sumac and toss well. In another bowl, beat the hummus with a little olive oil and seasoning. Add in some lime juice and harissa, if desired. Pour the seasoning over the salad and toss well. Garnish with mint.

Fun Facts

This recipe is an easy salad to whip up at any time, provided you have a can of chickpeas ready. Easy and wholesome, this salad is quite the dish!

91. Citrus Fish

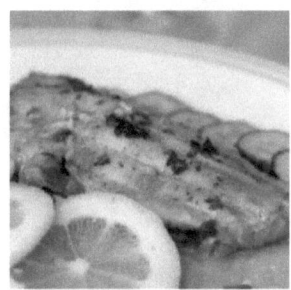

Summary

This buttery sauce with the lightly pan-fried fish, will have the children asking for another helping!

Ingredients

- 3-4 fillets of fish, John Dory or salmon
- ½ cup lemon juice
- 1 stick butter, halved
- Cornflour, if needed
- Salt and pepper
- Pinch of herbs
- Handful of parsley, chopped

Method

1. Season fish with salt and pepper and keep aside. Heat a skillet and add butter. First cook the fish fillets on it for about 2 minutes per side, and

transfer to a plate. Now add remaining butter to pan along with parsley, salt, pepper and heat. Take off gas, stir in the lemon juice and spoon over fish fillets. Serve with a side of boiled beans and mash if you like.

Fun Facts

The corn flour is added to ingredients, if you would like the sauce to be thicker in consistency.

92. Tomato Spiced Risotto

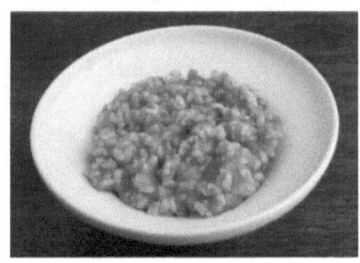

Summary

If your children love a good risotto, then try this variation with them!

Ingredients

- 1 tsp. fennel seeds
- 2 tomatoes, chopped fine
- Olive oil
- 2L Chicken stock or vegetable stock
- 1 packet Arborio rice
- 150ml white wine, for cooking
- 2 tbsp. finely grated parmesan
- 1 large onion, finely chopped
- 2-3 garlic cloves, finely minced

Method

1. Add olive oil to a skillet and sauté onion, garlic and add a pinch of seasoning. Meanwhile, heat stock in a separate pan on low heat. Now add rice to the pan and sauté for 2 minutes. Then add the wine, turn on the heat so it has the chance to evaporate yet leave a flavor.

2. Once wine is absorbed, add a spoonful of stock and stir till absorbed. Repeat this process until each time the stock is absorbed. Add tomatoes and fennel before your last two spoonful of stock. Serve with grated Parmesan.

Fun Facts

Remember to cook the risotto to al dente stage, where it is cooked but has a certain bite to the texture.

93. Pesto Pasta

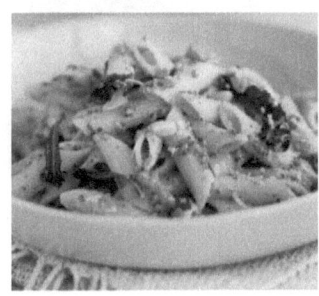

Summary

A quick meal for whenever you need it and when you can't think of whipping up something else.

Ingredients

- 100 g basil leaves
- 5 garlic cloves
- 1 cup extra virgin olive oil
- 2-3 tbsp. toasted pine nuts
- Grated parmesan cheese
- Salt and pepper
- 250g Fusilli pasta
- Handful of cooked chicken

Method

1. Add basil leaves, garlic, salt, olive oil, pine nuts and pepper to a grinder and pulse on high speed till you get a lovely green mixture. Then add in little parmesan cheese and give it a last blend.

2. Boil pasta according to instructions. add this to a pan along with the sauce, reserved pasta water, and cooked chicken at the last stage. Serve with basil leaves and grated Parmesan.

Fun Facts

Store the chicken and the pesto sauce in your freezer for use anytime. This is a quick meal that can be made within minutes for your hungry children!

94. Tenderloin with Salsa

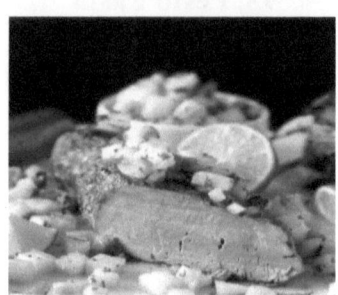

Summary

The mango salsa is sure to be a hit with your kids and everyone else at home! Make ahead and store in the fridge.

Ingredients

- 1 mango, chopped
- 2 scallions, chopped
- 1 tablespoon plus 1 teaspoon olive oil
- 1 tablespoon fresh lime juice
- 1/4 teaspoon crushed red pepper
- Kosher salt
- 1 1 1/4-pound pork tenderloin
- 1 teaspoon ground coriander

Method

1. Combine mango with scallions, oil, red pepper flakes, lime juice, salt and pepper. Rub the meat with oil, coriander leaves and seasoning. Broil the meat for about 15 minutes or until cooked. Slice and serve with mango salsa on top.

Fun Facts

Usually a salsa is a tomato based sauce but can be made with a variation of combining tomatoes with pineapple or mango.

95. Seriously Sloppy Joe's

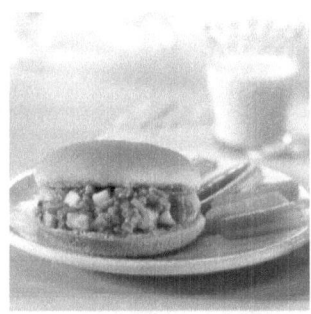

Summary

The more filling you add to the bun, the sloppier they get! On the same note, these contain a good amount of protein.

Ingredients

- 1 medium carrot, chopped fine
- 8-ounce lean ground beef
- 1 cup onion, chopped fine
- 2 teaspoon garlic powder
- ½ teaspoon chili powder
- 1/4 teaspoon black pepper
- 1/4 cup ketchup
- 1 tablespoon Worcestershire sauce
- 1 tablespoon Dijon mustard
- 1 teaspoon red wine vinegar
- 2 tablespoon tomato paste
- 1 can tomato sauce
- 8 hamburger buns

Method

1. Heat skillet and add carrot, onion, beef and cook until beef is browned and vegetables are cooked. Put garlic powder, chili powder and pepper. In bowl mix ketchup, tomato sauce, Worcestershire sauce, red

wine vinegar and tomato paste and pour into pan till it thickens. Once sauce is ready, add in between two lightly toasted burger buns and enjoy!

Fun Facts

Sloppy Joe's refers to a type of American burger and have been around since 1950s!

96. Pasta with Chunky Meat Sauce

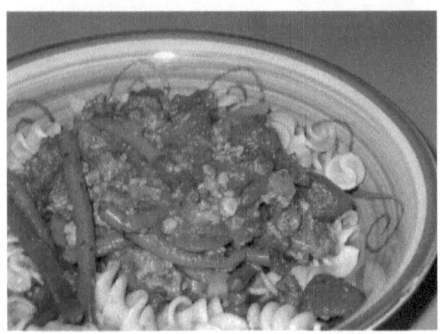

Summary

For those who like a chunky meat sauce, here's the dish for you!

Ingredients

- 1 packet fresh linguine
- 1/2-pound lean ground beef
- 1 cup finely chopped onion
- 2 tablespoon minced fresh garlic
- Pinch of dried oregano
- Salt, to taste
- 3-4 tablespoons tomato paste
- 1 can diced tomatoes
- 1/4 cup grated Parmesan cheese
- 2 tablespoon fresh flat-leaf parsley leaves

Method

1. Cook pasta according to relevant instructions. In another skillet heat the garlic and onion followed by oregano and salt and beef and cook

until beef is golden brown. Put in the tomato paste thereafter the tomatoes and boil. Follow suit with the pasta, cheese and parsley.

Fun Facts

There is huge difference in taste between freshly made pasta and store bought and packaged pasta! Try it for yourself, sometime!

97. Lamb and Veg Stew

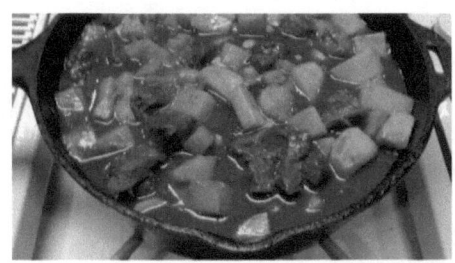

Summary

A stew is always considered to be comfort food. Try on your kids on a cold winter evening.

Ingredients

- 3 tablespoons olive oil
- 2 onions, sliced
- 2 pounds lamb steaks, bones removed and meat cut into 2-inch pieces
- Kosher salt and black pepper
- 3 carrots cut into 3-inch sticks
- 1/2 cup white wine
- 2.5 cups chicken broth
- 2 tablespoon all-purpose flour
- 1 cup fresh flat-leaf parsley, roughly chopped
- 1 can diced tomatoes, drained
- 1 cup green beans, chopped into tiny bits

Method

1. Season lamb and keep aside and heat a skillet with oil by the side. Cook it on the skillet and keep aside on a plate. Add remaining vegetables to the pot and cover and cook. Add flour and cook and then add wine. Follow it up with the broth, beans and tomatoes. Simmer

until lamb and vegetables are tender. Check for seasoning and serve with parsley.

Fun Facts

This stew can also be cooled to room temperature and frozen in a bag for up to a good 3 months!

98. Mushroom Soup with Barley

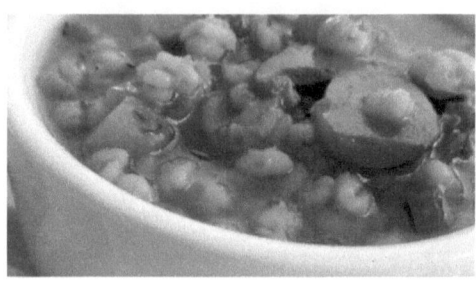

Summary

Let the soup remain chunky for added flavor, but it can also be pureed if your kids like a smooth soup.

Ingredients

- 3/4 cup pearl barley
- 3 packets mushrooms, sliced
- 3 cups carrots, chopped
- 3 tablespoons olive oil
- 3 sprigs fresh thyme
- Salt and black pepper
- 3 cloves garlic, sliced
- 6-7 cups vegetable broth
- 1 tablespoon chopped flat-leaf parsley, for garnish

Method

1. Heat a skillet with oil. Throw in garlic, mushrooms and thyme and let it cook till softens. Add the carrots in as well, as they take time to cook. Pour in the broth with barley and seasoning and cook on a slow simmer for a while. Serve with a garnish of parsley.

Fun Facts

Try using various mushrooms for this recipe like a mixed bunch for much more flavor!

99. Bean Soup with Sausages

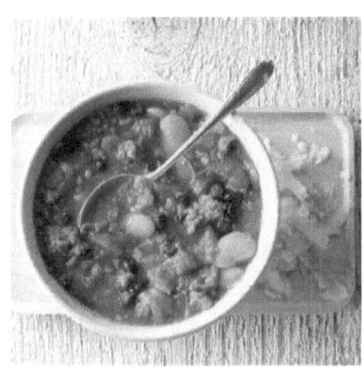

Summary

The beans add to the health quotient of this dish while the sausages add to the enhanced flavor.

Ingredients

- 1 cans cannellini beans, rinsed and slightly mashed
- 3/4th pound fully cooked chicken sausages, sliced
- 4 cloves garlic, sliced
- 3 tablespoons olive oil
- 6-7 cups chicken broth
- Salt and black pepper
- 1 small escarole head, torn

Method

1. Start by sautéing sausages in a pot followed by garlic and pinch of salt. Pour in broth, escarole, beans and seasoning. Cook till it is tender.

Fun Facts

The chicken sausages will emit a different flavor into the soup.

100. Fish with Tomato Olive Salsa

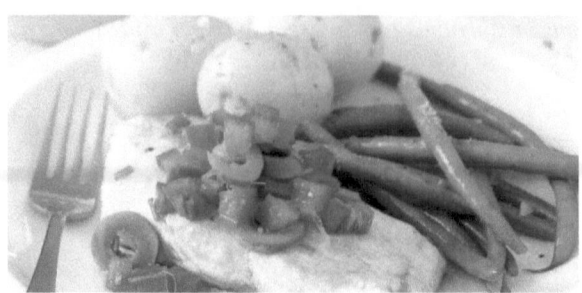

Summary

There is no reason needed to gorge on a piece of gorgeous healthy fish with a side of this tangy salsa.

Ingredients

- 3 tsp. olive oil
- Sea bass or John Dory fillets
- ½ cup dry white wine
- 1 onion, finely diced
- 1 cup diced tomatoes
- 3 tbsp. capers
- Red pepper flakes
- 2 cups spinach leaves
- ½ cup black olives
- Flour for dusting
- Salt and pepper

Method

1. Dust the fish with flour and salt and pat off excess. Cook it on a heated skillet for 2 minutes on each side. Keep aside. In the same pan, add onion and sauté. Pour in the wine and reduce. Add olives, tomatoes, caper and red chili flakes. Cook and add spinach till it wilts. Season and serve the salsa over the fried fish.

Fun Facts

If you like the strong flavor of capers, then this is a must have salsa with the fish.

101. Shrimp Noodle Soup

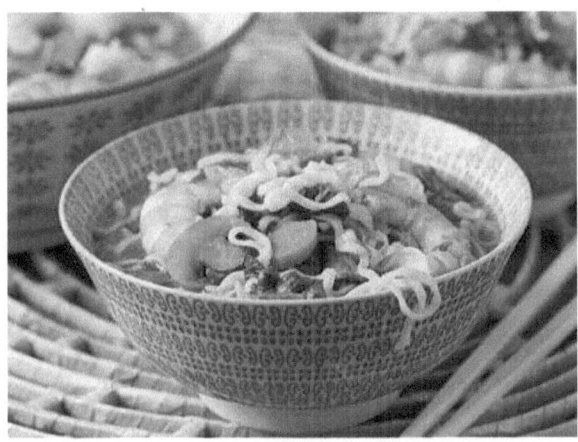

Summary

Shrimp and noodles is an ultimate combination in this Asian inspired soup!

Ingredients

- 1/2 red pepper, sliced
- 7 cups chicken broth
- 20-30-pound medium shrimp, peeled and deveined
- 1/4 small head Napa cabbage, chopped
- 3 tablespoons soy sauce
- 1 cup snow peas, halved
- Handful of basil leaves, shredded
- 1 tablespoon rice vinegar

Method

1. Heat broth, soy sauce and peppers in a large potful. Add the cabbage, followed by noodles and snow peas and vinegar. Just as it comes to a boil, throw in the shrimps. Serve with a smattering of basil leaves.

Fun Facts

Shrimps are an exclusive source of anti-oxidants and packed with anti-inflammatory nutrients so this dish becomes a healthy meal option.

102. Pesto Soup with Chickpeas

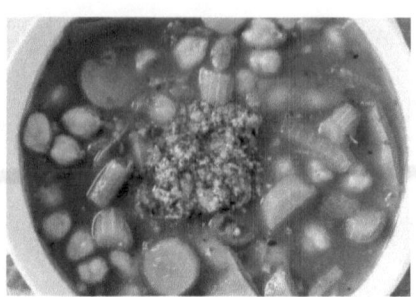

Summary

The unusual combination of pesto and chickpeas makes for a wholesome soup option.

Ingredients

- 1/2-pound green beans, halved
- 1 cup frozen peas
- 1 can chickpeas, rinsed
- 1/4 cup pesto
- 2 stalks celery, chopped
- 2 tablespoons olive oil
- 2 onions, chopped
- 3 carrots, sliced
- 3 tablespoons tomato paste
- Salt and black pepper
- 7 cups vegetable broth

Method

1. Heat oil in a skillet and add carrots, onions, celery and seasoning and cook till tender. Add in the tomato paste and let it cook for 2 minutes. Pour in broth, peas, beans and chickpeas and simmer till tender. Add in a dollop of pesto and turn off the heat. Let it rest and then ladle into bowls.

Fun Facts

Also known as garbanzo beans or ceci, this hails from the Middle Eastern region, and is a primary component of the hummus dish!

103. Chorizo Pea Soup

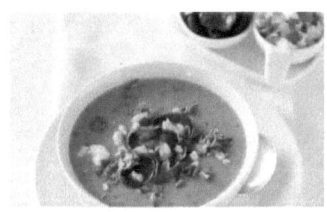

Summary

You can lure your kids to this soup on the basis of the wonderful chorizo in it! The health aspect present in the peas will follow suit.

Ingredients

- 5 ounces cured chorizo, chopped
- 2 small onion, chopped
- 8 cups chicken broth
- 1-2 cups split peas
- Salt and black pepper

Method

1. Sauté chorizo and brown it in a pot. To this oil, add onions to soften, chicken broth, seasoning and peas. Cover and cook till peas are tender.

Fun Facts

The chorizo releases enough fat to cook the onion and peas in, giving the dish a wonderful flavor!

104. Tomato Bruschetta's

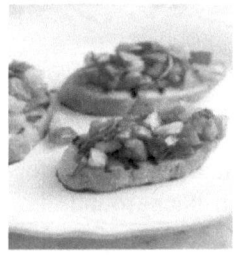

Summary

The classic bruschetta recipe which can be served alongside a soup, or even just gobbled up when really hungry!

Ingredients

- 3 tomatoes, chopped
- 3 cloves garlic minced
- 1 tsp. basil, finely chopped
- Extra virgin olive oil
- Salt and pepper
- 1 baguette, cut into slices
- Basil leaves, for garnish

Method

1. Mix the first five ingredients in a glass bowl and set aside till some juices are released. Spread this mixture over buttered and toasted slices of the baguette and garnish with basil leaves and enjoy!

Fun Facts

This recipe can be made even at short notice, or when you have sudden guests over.

105. Aubergine Sandwiches

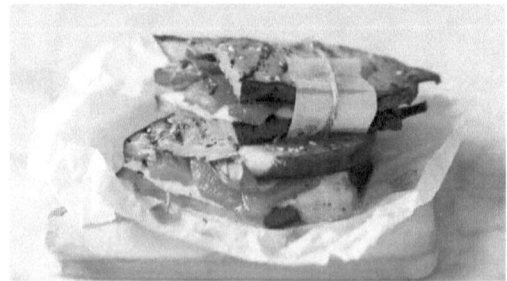

Summary

This aubergine filling is an unusual filling for a sandwich, and is possibly inspired from a Mediterranean background. This stays well in the fridge for about a week.

Ingredients

- 2 large aubergines, peeled, sliced and salted
- 2-3 cloves of garlic
- Juice of 1 lemon
- 4-5 tbsp. extra virgin olive oil
- Handful mint leaves, roughly chopped
- Slices of bread

Method

1. Take a large bowl and mix first 5 ingredients thoroughly. Your filling is now ready. Add it amidst two slices of bread, like a sandwich and grill it. Your sandwich is now ready!

Fun Facts

Aubergines have different names and are also known as brinjals or eggplants depending on the region you hail from!

106. Chicken Burritos

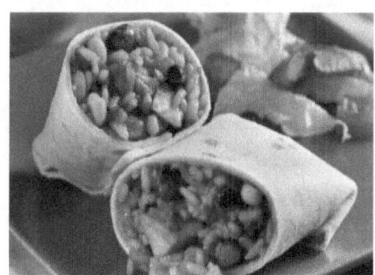

Summary

Mexican inspired dishes are always a pleasure to make for children as they are very easy, loved by most kids and a wholesome meal too.

Ingredients

- 2-4 flour tortillas, available at store
- 1 onion, finely chopped
- pound tender chicken breast, cut into 1-inch pieces
- 1 teaspoons chili powder
- 1 can black beans, rinsed and drained

- 1/2 teaspoon ground cumin
- 2 teaspoons oil
- Salt and pepper
- 2 garlic cloves, minced
- 1/4 cup Monterey Jack cheese or any other
- 1/4 cup reduced-fat sour cream
- pico de gallo

Method

1. Add onion, garlic, meat, chili and cumin powder salt and pepper to a hot skillet and cook chicken through. Add beans and sauté for 2 minutes. Toast the tortillas on a pan first. Then spoon the mixture into tortillas and fold in. Your burritos are ready to be served with a dollop of sour cream and pico de gallo.

Fun Facts

Burritos are a good way to pack nutrients into your child's stomach, all in one roll.

107. British Fish and Chips

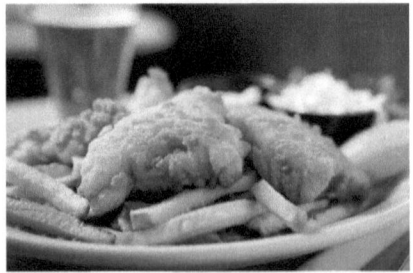

Summary

This crispy crunchy fish is surely going to be a hot with the children of the family!

Ingredients

- 4 John Dory fillets
- 2 tsp. mayonnaise
- 1 large packet potato chips, crushed
- Salt and pepper

- ½ cup ranch dressing
- ½ tsp. finely pressed garlic, mixed into

Method

1. Preheat the oven to the highest temperature. Add fish fillets on a lined sheet. Brush with salt and pepper and the mayonnaise. Crush the potato chips and sprinkle over each fillet. Cook for about 10 minutes or till fish is cooked through. Serve with ranch and garlic dressing.

Fun Facts

To think that Fish and Chips existed in Britain for 150 years and have survived through both the World Wars!

108. BBQ Chicken Sandwich

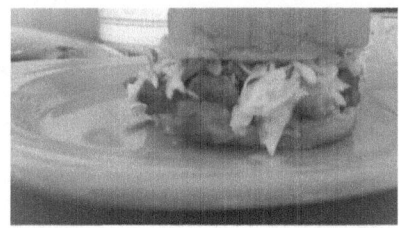

Summary

This sweet spicy sandwich recipe is a hot favorite with any kid!

Ingredients

- 2 cups barbecue sauce
- 1/4 cup pickled jalapeños, roughly chopped (optional)
- 5 cups rotisserie chicken, meat shredded
- Lime juice, if desired
- Potato fries (optional)
- 4 whole wheat hamburger buns

Method

1. Mix together BBQ sauce, shredded chicken and jalapenos. Squeeze in a little lime, if you desire. Add this filling into burger buns and serve with a side portion of fries.

Fun Facts

Burger and fries have become a like a married couple! You can't seem to have one without the other!

109. Tuna and Caper Sandwich

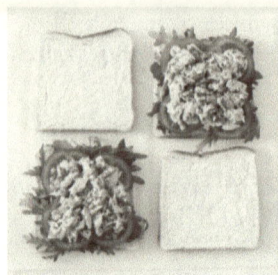

Summary

Tuna and capers form a good combination, and this tangy mix for the sandwiches is a good change from the regular fillings.

Ingredients

- 2 6-ounce cans of tuna packed in water (drained)
- 1 tablespoon extra-virgin olive oil
- 1/4 teaspoon black pepper
- 1/2 cup fresh flat-leaf parsley, roughly chopped
- 1 tablespoon capers, roughly chopped
- 1 teaspoon lemon zest
- 2 teaspoons lemon juice
- 8 slices sandwich bread

Method

1. Add the 1st seven ingredients to a bowl and mix thoroughly. This is your filling for sandwiches are ready. Spread it on a slice of bread and cover with the top slice and enjoy.

Fun Facts

Did you know that tuna is amongst the fish that is considered a superfood due to its Omega 3 fatty acids?

110. Creamy Zucchini Pasta

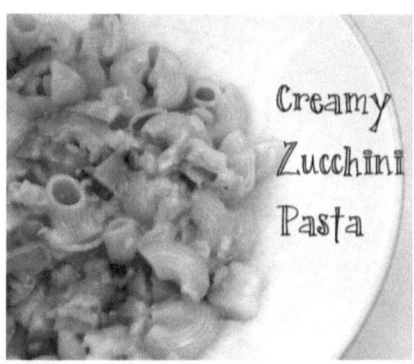

Summary

This colorful green pasta is wonderfully creamy with the addition of the healthy avocado.

Ingredients

- 1 large zucchini, sliced into spirals
- 1 Roma tomato or regular tomato
- ½ an avocado
- 2 cloves garlic, roughly chopped
- 1 tsp. olive oil
- 2 tsp. lime juice
- 1 tsp. dried basil or oregano
- 1 tbsp. chopped and toasted walnuts
- Water, optional

Method

1. Drop zucchini spirals into boiling water and remove immediately and keep aside. Add chopped tomatoes to it as well. In a bowl, add parsley, lime juice, garlic, olive oil, basil and water along with a smattering of walnuts and pulse in a blender. Use this sauce to toss your zucchini noodles in.

Fun Facts

While these looks exactly like a green version of noodles, they are in fact made of zucchini or courgettes and are thus a healthier option.

111. Pork with Cabbage Noodles

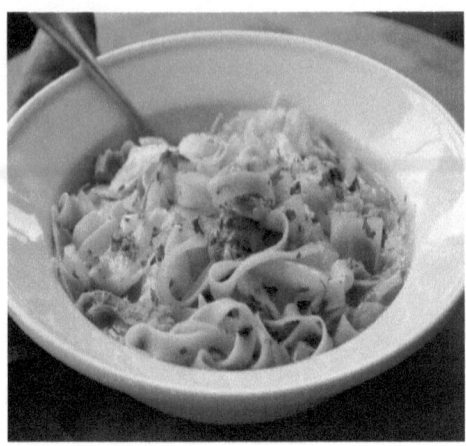

Summary

Cabbage is one of the vegetables that don't go down very easily with kids and adults alike. Convert them with these noodles and be amazed at how fast they are gobbled down!

Ingredients

- 1 tbsp. coconut oil
- ¾ lb. pork mince
- 1 lb. cabbage, spiral sliced
- 1 onion, finely chopped
- 1 tbsp. ginger, grated
- 2 tbsp. garlic powder
- 1 green onions, bunch
- 1 tbsp. fish sauce
- Juice of ½ lime
- 1 tbsp. dried or fresh basil
- 12-15 mint leaves, chopped roughly

Method

1. Slice cabbage and onion and keep aside. Side by side, chop green onion, mint and cilantro. Heat a large skillet, add coconut oil and throw in garlic, ginger, fish sauce. Fry until crisp and keep aside once done.

2. Add pork with remaining ginger-garlic sauce and cook till done. Add the other mixture too and garnish with cilantro and mint leaves and spring onions. Add a tad bit of lime before serving.

Fun Facts

Include a few tips here about the dish, or include a few fun facts about some of the ingredients. For example, if the main ingredient in this recipe was broccoli, write the title "3 Reasons Broccoli Helps Reduce Cholesterol", and then just write down the 3 reasons.

112. Thai Soup

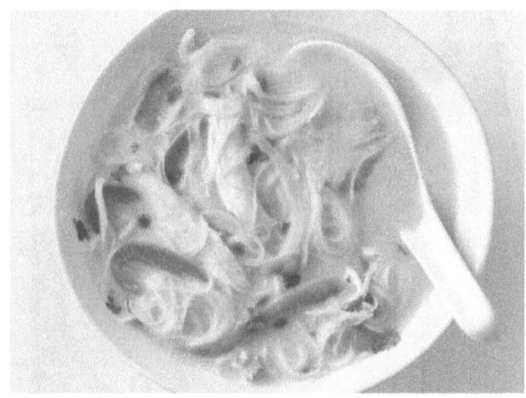

Summary

This Thai inspired Asian soup with squash is an unusual soup which will be loved by one and all.

Ingredients

- 2 small white onion, chopped
- 1 butternut squash, peeled and cut into 1-inch pieces
- Salt
- 2 tablespoons olive oil
- 4 cups chicken broth
- 2-3 tablespoons Thai green curry paste
- 1 can coconut milk
- 1 tablespoons lime juice
- Chili-garlic sauce, optional

Method

1. Cook onion in a skillet with oil on medium heat with salt, curry paste, stock, coconut milk and butternut squash. Simmer till tender. Turn off the heat and add in lime juice. Add a dollop of chili-garlic sauce if you wish.

Fun Facts

In the recent years, coconut milk has received a great deal of attention due to its health benefits and has been majorly popularized around the world.

113. Cauliflower Soup

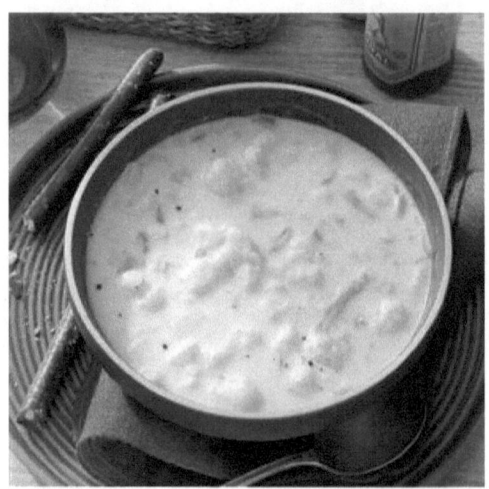

Summary

Write a little about why this dish is healthy and helps with the proposed solution. Maybe address one or two of the key ingredients.

Ingredients

- 4 cloves garlic, sliced
- 2-3 tablespoons olive oil
- 1 medium cauliflower, chopped
- 2 tsp. thyme leaves
- 6 cups chicken broth
- Salt and black pepper

Method

1. First cook garlic till golden brown. Add cauliflower florets, thyme, stock, salt and pepper and simmer. Blitz the soup till smooth retaining some cauliflower florets to munch on! Garnish with garlic and olive oil and a sprig of thyme.

Fun Facts

Did you know that a cauliflower is actually a flower species that hasn't fully developed?!

114. Apple Cheese Sandwiches

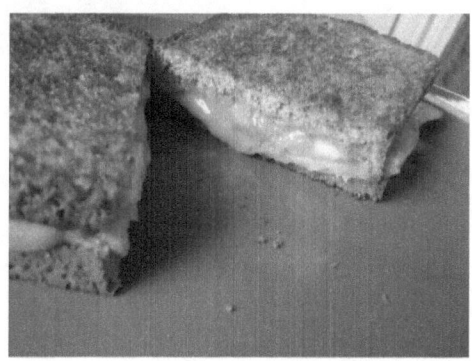

Summary

Apple and a strong cheese have an unusual flavor combination that go well together. For children, try and use a milder cheese.

Ingredients

- 1 teaspoon whole-grain mustard or Dijon mustard
- 1 ounce thinly sliced Cheddar or any strong cheese
- 1 whole apple, thinly sliced
- 2-4 slices of multi grain bread

Method

1. Butter the bread. Top it with the mustard spread. Fill one side of the sandwich with apple slices and the other with the cheese slice. Close up and enjoy!

Fun Facts

If you are bored of your regular sandwiches, here's an option for something different!

115. Sambal Chicken Sandwiches

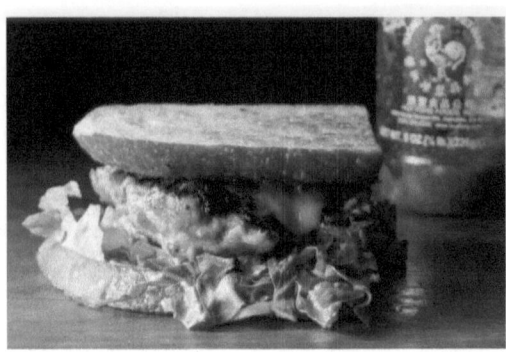

Summary

This Malaysian inspired chicken filling is a great option for a family meal. It can be paired with a slightly bland soup to ease out the spice.

Ingredients

- 2 tbsp. sambal oelek sauce
- 1 cup shredded chicken
- Salt and pepper
- Juice of half a lime

Method

1. In a bowl, combine chicken with the sambal sauce, seasoning and a squeeze of lime juice. Use this as filling to form sandwiches.

Fun Facts

You can add a slice of cheese if the filling proves to be too spicy to handle.

116. Pesto Tuna Subway

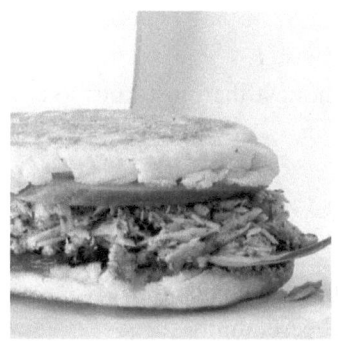

Summary

Tuna is a healthy fish releasing healthy Omega 3 fatty acids while the tuna contains healthy pine nuts.

Ingredients

- 2 cans of tuna packed in water (drained)
- 1/4 teaspoon black pepper
- 4 heaped tablespoons store-bought pesto
- 3-4 subway bread rolls

Method

1. Add all the ingredients except the bread to a bowl and mix well. Use this as a filing for your sandwiches.

Fun Facts

This mixture even stays well in the fridge for a good one week.

117. Egg and Prosciutto Panini

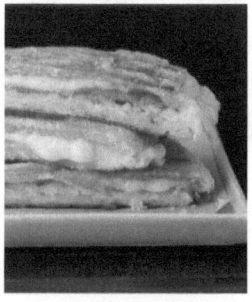

Summary

Eggs are proved to be amongst the most nutritious food options available on this planet!

Ingredients

- 10 large eggs
- Kosher salt and black pepper
- 8 ounces Swiss cheese, thinly sliced
- 10 ounces prosciutto, thinly sliced
- 4 soft rolls, halved lengthwise
- 4 tablespoons unsalted butter

Method

1. Add eggs, seasoning and mix together. In a hot skillet, add butter and scramble eggs and place straight on the bottom of the sandwich. Layer with prosciutto and cheese and basil leaves if you wish. Enjoy these hot!

Fun Facts

This sandwich is a killer combination and works well all the time.

118. Chicken Noodles

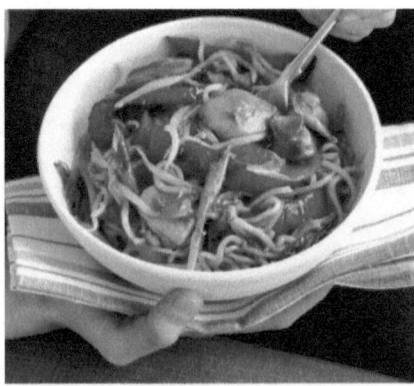

Summary

Super-fast and very kid friendly, this recipe is loaded with vegetables.

Ingredients

- 4 garlic cloves, crushed
- Fresh ginger root, grated
- 1 red chilli, deseeded and chopped
- 3 packs dried egg noodles
- 2 tbsp. soy sauce
- 2 tbsp. tomato purée
- 2 chicken breasts, cut into chunky strips
- 1 small broccoli, broken into florets
- 2 carrots, cut into thin sticks
- 1 large pack beansprouts
- 1 tbsp. vegetable oil
- 1 tbsp. oyster sauce, mixed in 2 tbsp. of water
- 3 spring onions, halved and sliced into long strips

Method

1. Combine chili, ginger, garlic, soy sauce and tomato puree in a bowl and use as marinade for chicken. Boil egg noodles along with carrots and broccoli. Heat a large wok, add chicken along with the marinade, noodles, vegetables, bean sprouts and toss. Then mix in oyster sauce into it.

Fun Facts

The longer you keep the chicken marinating, the more flavor it will acquire.

119. Peas Pasta

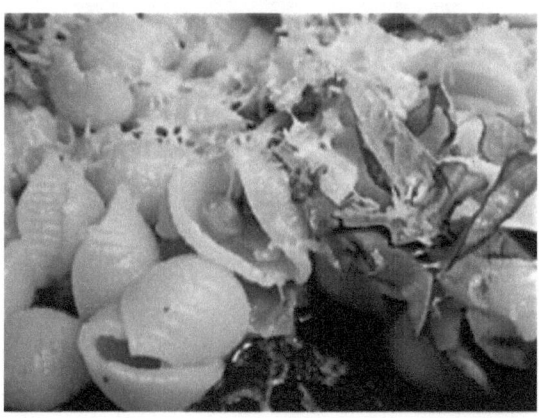

Summary

A good way to get peas down your child's throat is to mix it up with their favorite meal- pasta!

Ingredients

- 1 small packet frozen peas
- 1 packet mixed pasta shapes
- 200g piece of cooked chicken, chopped into cubes
- 1 tbsp. creamed wasabi mixed with 1 tbsp. cream
- Salt and ground black pepper
- 3 tbsp. roughly chopped parsley

Method

1. Cook pasta according to instructions. just before you turn off the heat, add the peas and drain. In a skillet, add chicken, wasabi mixture and parsley and cook with salt and pepper. Stir in the pasta when chicken is done, and serve into bowls.

Fun Facts

The different pasta shapes itself will attract children to the pasta making it a successful meal idea.

120. Simple Chocolate Cheesecake

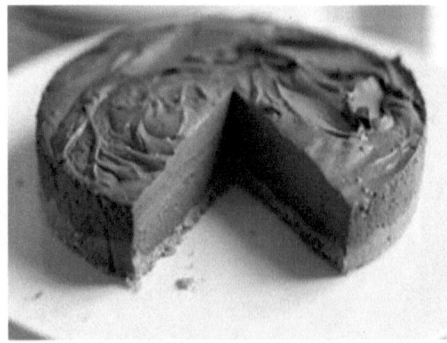

Summary

A good meal always needs a better dessert to end with! So here it is!

Ingredients

- 300g soft cream cheese
- A packet of digestive biscuits, crushed
- 200g mascarpone cheese
- 80g-100g melted butter
- 300g milk chocolate
- 100g dark chocolate

Method

1. Take a bowl and mix mascarpone with cream cheese. In another bowl mix biscuits with melted butter, and then use this to form a base of the baking tin. Add milk to the cheese mixture and then stir in both of the melted chocolates. Pour into the tin and refrigerate for over 2 hours.

Fun Facts

A cheesecake has a wonderfully creamy texture that leaves a lasting impression on your tongue!

121. Garden Pasta Salad

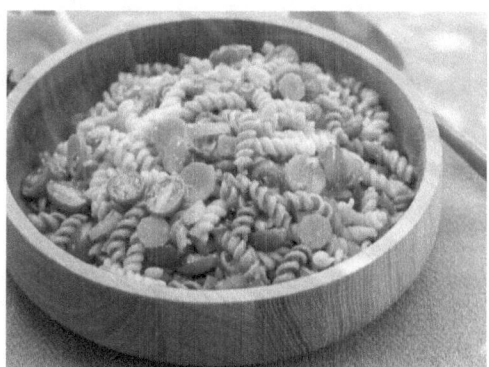

Ingredients

- 2 package (16 ounce each) tri-color spiral pasta, cook according to instructions on the package
- 1 cup carrots, thinly sliced
- 4 stalks celery, chopped
- 1 cup green bell pepper, chopped
- 1 cup cucumber, peeled, thinly sliced

- 4 large tomatoes, chopped
- ½ cup onions, chopped
- 4 bottles (16 ounce each) Italian style salad dressing
- 1 cup parmesan cheese, grated

Method

1. Add all the ingredients except the dressing and cheese to a large bowl and toss. Pour the dressing and cheese and toss well. Chill for an hour and serve.

122. Texas Coleslaw

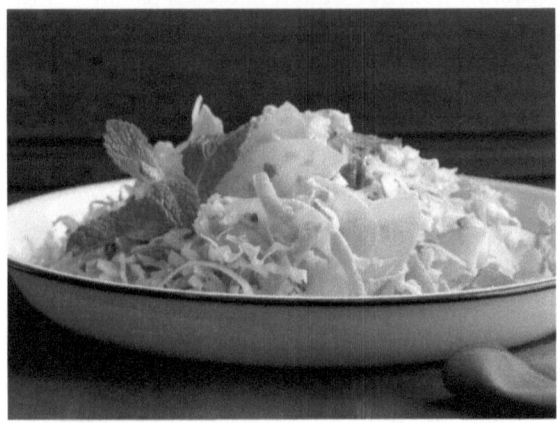

Ingredients

- 2 cups mayonnaise
- 2 tablespoons lime juice
- 2 tablespoons ground cumin
- 2 teaspoons salt
- Pepper powder to taste
- 1 large head cabbage, thinly sliced
- 2 large carrots, peeled, shredded
- 4 green onions, sliced
- 4 radishes, sliced

Method

1. Mix together all the ingredients in a bowl and refrigerate until use.

123. Potato Salad

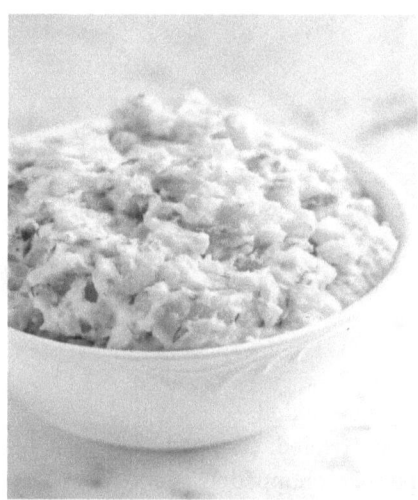

Ingredients

- ½ pound potatoes (red or new), scrubbed
- ½ pound fava bean pods, shelled
- 1 fennel bulb, thinly sliced
- 1 tablespoon fennel fronds
- 1 tablespoons chives, chopped
- 1 ½ tablespoons extra virgin olive oil
- ½ tablespoon lemon juice
- ½ teaspoon lemon zest
- Salt to taste
- Freshly ground pepper to taste

Method

1. Boil potatoes in a large pot of water with salt added to it. Drain and keep aside to cool. Blanch the fava beans in boiling water for about ½ a minute. Drain and transfer into a bowl of chilled water. Drain the beans and remove the skin of the beans. Chop the potatoes into bite sized pieces and place in a bowl.

2. In a small bowl, add olive oil, lemon juice, zest and whisk well. Pour over the potatoes and toss well. Add rest of the ingredients, salt, and pepper and mix well. Can serve as it is or chilled.

124. Picnic Summer Slaw

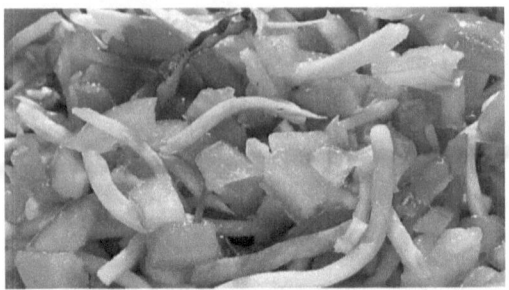

Ingredients

- 5-ounce cabbage, shredded
- 1 small cucumber, peeled, chopped
- ½ green bell pepper, chopped
- 1 medium tomato, peeled, chopped
- 2 green onions, sliced
- ¼ cup sugar
- ¼ cup vegetable oil
- 2 tablespoons white vinegar
- Salt to taste
- Pepper powder to taste

Method

1. Mix together in a small saucepan sugar, oil, vinegar, salt, and pepper. Place the saucepan over medium heat. Cook until the sugar is melted. Cool. Mix together rest of the ingredients in a bowl and pour the cooled dressing. Toss and refrigerate for a couple of hours.

125. Sweet Corn and Tomato Salad

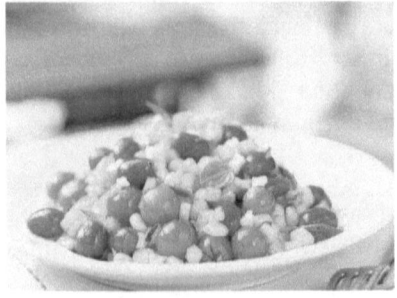

Ingredients

- 2 medium ripe tomatoes, seeded, roughly chopped, pat dried
- 3 ears fresh sweet corn, shucked
- 2 tablespoons fresh mint leaves, minced
- 2 tablespoons fresh mixed herbs of your choice, minced
- ½ tablespoon olive oil
- Kosher salt to taste
- Freshly ground black pepper to taste
- 2-ounce soft goat cheese, chilled, crumbled

Method

1. Place a pot of water over medium heat. Add corn and boil for 5-6 minutes. Drain the water and keep aside to cool. When cooled, remove the corn kernels off the cob with a knife. Mix together corn and tomatoes in a bowl. Add the herbs, salt, pepper, cheese, and toss. Serve immediately.

126. Pork Tenderloin and Cucumber Salad

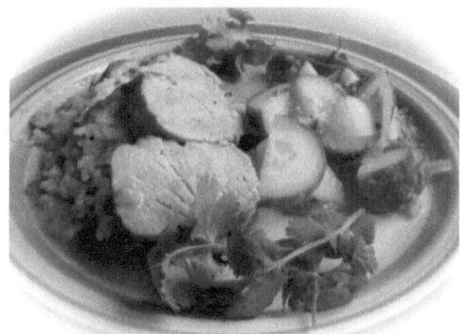

Ingredients

- 2 tablespoons extra virgin olive oil + extra for grilling and rubbing
- 1 teaspoon black pepper powder
- ¼ teaspoon white pepper powder
- ¼ teaspoon cayenne pepper
- Kosher salt to taste
- 1 pork tenderloin (about 1 ½ pounds), butter flied, lightly pounded
- 1 tablespoon fresh lime juice
- 1 tablespoon minced shallots
- 1 medium peach, diced

- ½ pound Persian cucumber, diced
- ¼ cup mint, chopped
- ¼ cup cilantro, chopped
- Plain yogurt to serve

Method

1. Grease a grill pan. Preheat a grill. Mix together in a bowl all the 3 peppers and salt. Rub olive oil all over the pork. Season with the pepper mixture.

2. Place the pork on the grill pan and grill until done. When cool, slice the pork. In a large bowl, add all the ingredients including pork except the yogurt and mix well. Serve with yogurt.

127. Great American Potato Salad

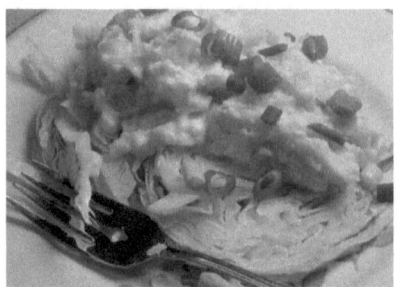

Ingredients

- ¼ cup mayonnaise
- ½ tablespoon yellow mustard
- ¼ teaspoon celery seed
- Pepper powder to taste
- ¾ pound potatoes
- 1 hardboiled egg, chopped
- 1 stalk celery, sliced
- 3 tablespoons dill pickle relish

Method

1. Mix together in a bowl, mayonnaise, mustard, celery and pepper powder. Add the remaining ingredients and mix well. Chill for a couple of hours before serving.

128. Olive Caprese Salad

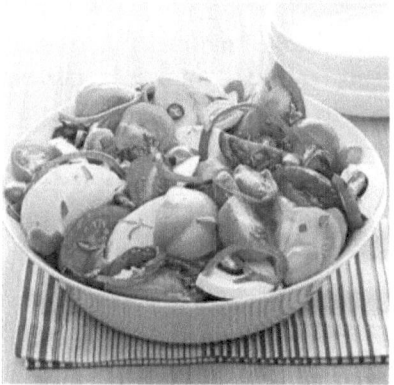

Ingredients

- ¾ cup red wine vinegar, divided
- ¼ cup sugar
- ½ a star anise
- 1 small red onion, sliced
- pound medium heirloom tomatoes, cut into wedges
- 1 cup heirloom cherry tomatoes, halved
- ½ cup pitted green olives, halved
- 4 ounces fresh mozzarella cheese, sliced, halved
- ½ tablespoon fresh basil, minced
- ½ tablespoon tarragon, minced
- ½ tablespoon mint, minced
- ½ tablespoon cilantro, minced
- 1 Serrano pepper, thinly sliced (optional)
- 2 tablespoons olive oil
- 1 tablespoon lime juice
- ¾ teaspoon lime zest, grated
- Salt to taste

Method

1. Mix together in a saucepan half the vinegar, sugar, and star anise. Place the saucepan over medium heat and boil until the sugar dissolves. Switch off the heat. After about 15 minutes, add onions and keep aside for half an hour. Discard the star anise. Drain the onions and retain about 2 tablespoons of the marinade. In a large bowl, add

the drained onions, tomatoes, olives, cheese, all the fresh herbs, and pepper.

2. In a small bowl, add oil, lime juice, the remaining vinegar, and zest. Whisk well. Pour over the tomatoes mixture. Add salt and toss. Sprinkle some of the retained marinade and serve.

129. Cheese Burger Bites

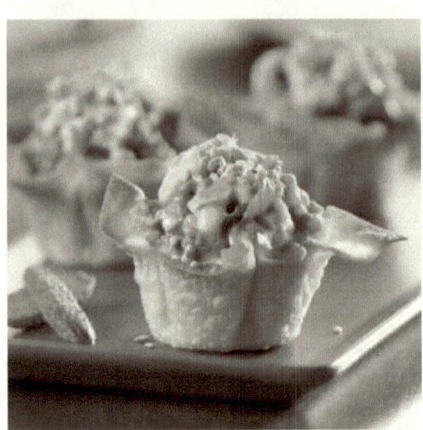

Ingredients

- 2 egg yolks, beaten
- pound lean ground beef
- ¼ cup onions, grated
- 1 teaspoon salt
- ¼ teaspoon pepper powder
- 12 slices bread, remove the crusts
- Cheddar cheese, grated

Method

1. Mix together egg yolk, beef, onions, salt, and pepper. Using your hands, make small balls of the mixture. Make small rounds of the bread with a cookie cutter (about 1 ½ inch rounds).

2. Place a meat ball on a round. Make a small well in the ball and fill with a little cheddar cheese. Place on a baking sheet. Repeat with the remaining meat balls and bread. Broil in a preheated oven for about 4-5 minutes. Garnish with green onions and serve with ketchup.

130. Spicy Peanuts

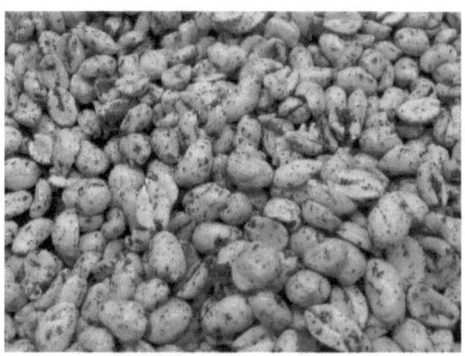

Ingredients

- 32-ounce unsalted, dry roasted peanuts
- ¼ cup canola oil
- 2 tablespoons sugar
- 3 teaspoons ground cumin
- 2 teaspoons salt
- 1 teaspoon cayenne pepper
- 1 teaspoon garlic powder

Method

1. Add all the ingredients to a bowl and toss well. Transfer the peanuts into a baking pan. Bake in a preheated oven at 300-degree F for about 20-25 minutes. Stir in between a couple of times. Cool completely and store in an air tight container.

131. Grilled Vegetable Skewers with Pesto Vinaigrette

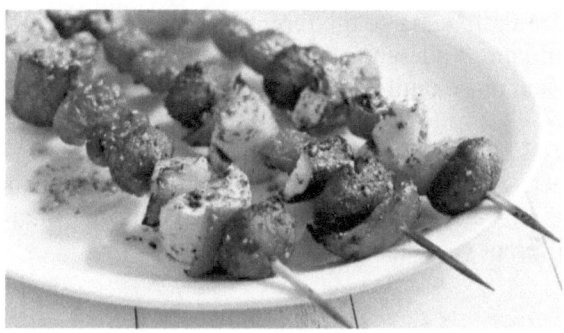

Ingredients

For Vinaigrette

- ¼ cup olive oil
- 2 -3 tablespoons pesto
- 1 tablespoon lemon juice

Vegetables for grilling

- 1/4-pound okra, stems removed
- 4 ounces mushrooms
- 1 bell pepper, seeded, cut into 1 ½ inch cubes
- 1 onion, cut into 1 ½ inch cubes
- 3 small summer squash, cut into 2 inch chunks
- ½ cup cherry tomatoes
- Sea salt to taste
- Freshly ground black pepper to taste

For the Pesto

- 1 cup packed fresh basil leaves
- 2 cloves garlic, minced
- 2 tablespoons pine nuts
- 1/3 cup extra virgin olive oil, divided
- Salt to taste
- Pepper powder to taste
- ¼ cup pecorino cheese, grated

Method

1. To make pesto: Place basil, garlic, and pine nuts in a food processor and pulse until a coarse mixture is formed. Add half the oil and blend until smooth. Add salt, pepper, remaining oil and pulse again. Add cheese and pulse until smooth.

2. For the Vinaigrette: Whisk together all the ingredients of vinaigrette and keep aside. For grilling vegetables: First soak the wooden skewers in water. Thread the vegetables on to the skewers alternating with different vegetables.

3. Brush the vegetables with the vinaigrette. Sprinkle salt and pepper over the vegetables. Grill on a preheated grill until the vegetables are done. Turn the skewers around in between. Serve with the vinaigrette.

132. Grilled Zucchini Rolls with Bacon and Cheese

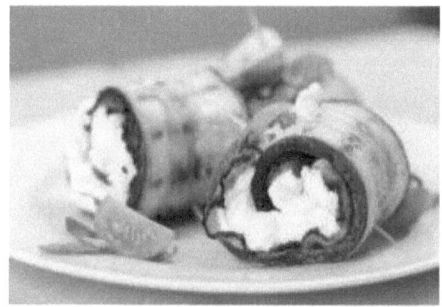

Ingredients

- 2 large zucchinis, sliced lengthwise into long slices
- ½ block cream cheese
- 5-6 strips of bacon
- 5-6 toothpicks

Method

1. Place the zucchini slices on a cookie sheet next to each other. Lay a piece of bacon on top of each zucchini slice. Smear a thin layer of cream cheese over each slice of bacon. Roll up a zucchini slice and fasten with a toothpick. Repeat with all the slices. Grill the zucchini rolls until the zucchini and bacon is cooked. When done, cool slightly and then serve.

133. Seven Layer Dip

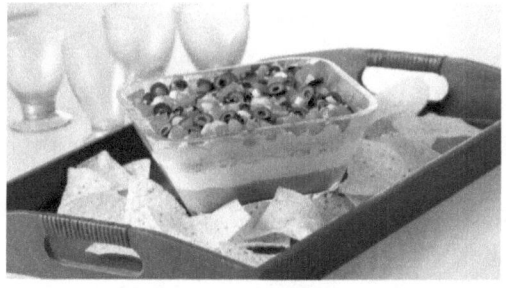

Ingredients

- 8 ounce canned refried beans
- ½ package taco seasoning
- ½ cup guacamole
- 4-ounce sour cream
- ½ cup chunky salsa or Pico de Gallo
- ½ cup cheddar cheese, shredded
- 1 Roma tomato, diced
- 2-3 green onions, chopped
- 1.25 ounce canned, sliced olives, drained
- 4 plastic tumblers
- Tortilla chips to serve

Method

1. Add refried beans and taco seasoning to a bowl and mix well. Divide the ingredients among the tumblers. Layer as follow: Bottom – refried beans. Next – sour cream. Next – guacamole. Next – salsa followed by cheese. Next – tomatoes. Top – green onions and olives. Garnish with a tortilla chip each and refrigerate. Serve!

134. Italian Skewers

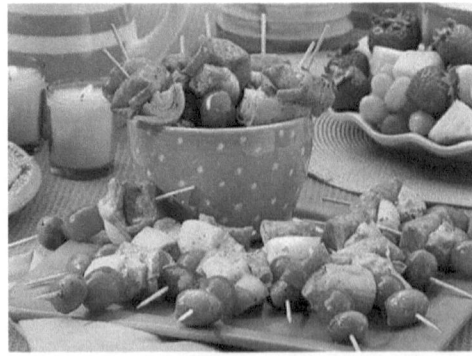

Ingredients

- 4-ounce block mozzarella cheese, chopped into 8 cubes
- 8 Genoa salami slices
- ½ a 14 ounce can small artichoke hearts, drained, halved
- ½ pint grape tomatoes
- ½ 6-ounce jar large Spanish olives, pitted, drained

- 8 wooden skewers
- ½ a 16-ounce bottle balsamic basil vinaigrette
- 1 tablespoon fresh lemon juice

Method

1. Place a cube of cheese each on the salami slice and wrap the cheese. Thread it on to the wooden skewers. Alternate with artichoke hearts, tomatoes, and olives. Place the skewers on a baking dish.

2. Mix together vinaigrette and lemon juice. Pour this mixture over the ready skewers. Cover and marinate for 8 hours in the refrigerator. Remove the skewers from the marinade and serve. Discard the remaining marinade.

135. Cornmeal Tarts with Cheese

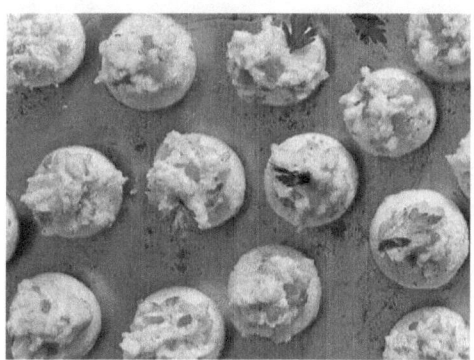

Ingredients

- 1 cup self-raising white cornmeal mix
- 1 cup buttermilk
- ¼ cup all-purpose flour
- 1 large, lightly beaten
- 2 tablespoons butter, melted
- 1 tablespoon sugar
- Ricotta pimiento cheese as much as you need

Method

1. Mix together in a large bowl all the ingredients except cheese. Grease mini muffin moulds. Pour this batter up to 2/3 full. Bake in a preheated oven at 400-degree F for about 15 minutes or until it is

golden brown. Scoop out about a teaspoon of the top of each muffin. Fill this with ricotta cheese and bake for 3-4 minutes until the cheese melts.

136. Sesame Salmon Croquettes

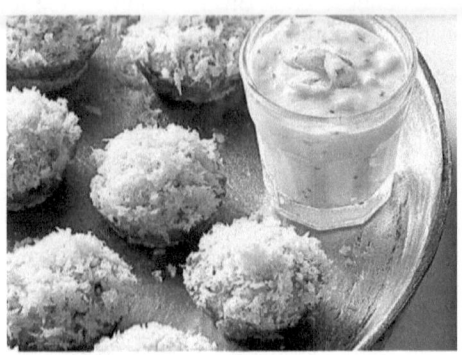

Ingredients

- 1 ¼ cups panko (Japanese breadcrumbs), divided
- 1 large egg
- 1 green onion, thinly sliced
- 2 tablespoons chopped fresh cilantro
- 2 tablespoons mayonnaise
- 1 teaspoon lime zest, grated
- 1 tablespoon fresh lime juice
- ½ tablespoon ginger, grated
- ½ a jar (1.62 ounce) sesame seeds, toasted
- 2 cloves garlic, minced
- ¼ teaspoon freshly ground pepper
- 3 tablespoons butter, melted
- Juice of ½ a lemon; retain the lemon after juicing it
- 1 tablespoon kosher salt
- ½ pound salmon fillet (chopped into 2- optional)

Method

1. Place together in a saucepan, lemon half, lemon juice, 1 tablespoon salt and 3 cups water. Place the saucepan over medium heat and bring to a boil. Add salmon, cover, lower heat and cook for about 4-5 minutes. (do not overcook it).

2. Remove the salmon with a slotted spoon and place in a bowl. When it cools, discard the skin and flake the salmon with a fork. Add half the panko and rest of the ingredients except butter and mix well. In a small bowl, mix together the remaining panko and butter. Grease muffin moulds. Add a teaspoon of this panko-butter mixture to each of the molds. Add 1 tablespoon of the salmon mixture over the panko mixture in each of the molds.

3. Add again a teaspoon of the panko mixture over the salmon in each of the molds. Place in a preheated oven at 425-degree F for 10 minutes or until the topmost panko mixture is golden brown. Serve warm with ginger Rémoulade.

137. Deviled Eggs

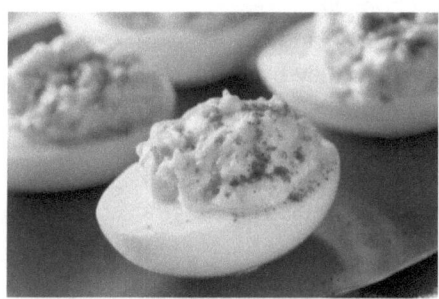

Ingredients

- 6 hardboiled eggs, peeled, halved lengthwise
- ¼ cup light mayonnaise
- 2 tablespoons prepared mustard
- 2 tablespoons apple cider vinegar
- ½ teaspoon sugar
- 3 tablespoons softened cream cheese
- 2 teaspoons fresh dill, chopped + extra for garnishing
- 1/8 teaspoon paprika

Method

1. Remove the yolks from the eggs and mash it and place it in a bowl. Add mayonnaise, mustard, vinegar, sugar, cream cheese, and dill. Mix well until smooth. Stuff the yolk cavity with this mixture. Refrigerate for a couple of hours. Sprinkle paprika and dill before serving.

138. Rancho Baked Beans

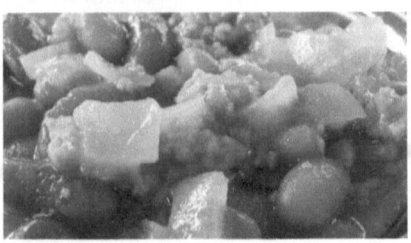

Ingredients

- ½ pound ground beef
- Cooking spray
- 1 cup onions, chopped
- 1 can (16 ounce) pork and beans
- ½ a 16 ounce can kidney beans, drained
- ½ cup ketchup
- 6 tablespoons brown sugar
- 1 tablespoon mustard
- ½ tablespoon white vinegar
- ½ teaspoon salt

Method

1. Place a skillet over medium heat. Add beef and onions. Sauté until the beef is browned. Remove with a slotted spoon, place in a large bowl, and discard the fat. Add rest of the ingredients to the bowl and mix well.

2. Spray a casserole dish with cooking spray. Transfer the entire contents of the bowl to the dish. Bake in a preheated oven at 350-degree F for about 45 minutes or until done.

139. Mexican Corn Bread

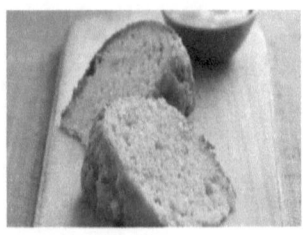

Ingredients

- ½ cup white sugar
- 2 eggs
- ½ a 15 ounce can cream style corn
- 2 ounces canned, chopped green chilli peppers, drained
- ¼ cup Monterey Jack cheese, shredded
- ½ cup all-purpose flour
- ½ cup yellow cornmeal
- 2 teaspoons baking powder
- ¼ teaspoon salt or to taste
- ¼ cup cheddar cheese

Method

1. In a large bowl, add butter and sugar. Beat well. Add egg and beat again. Add cream style corn, chilies, and cheeses. Mix well. In another bowl, mix together corn meal, flour, baking powder and salt. Add this to the cheese mixture. Mix well until smooth. Pour the batter into a greased baking dish.

2. Bake in a preheated oven at 300-degree F for about an hour or until a toothpick when inserted in the center of the dish comes out clean. Cool, slice and serve.

140. Baconista Brats

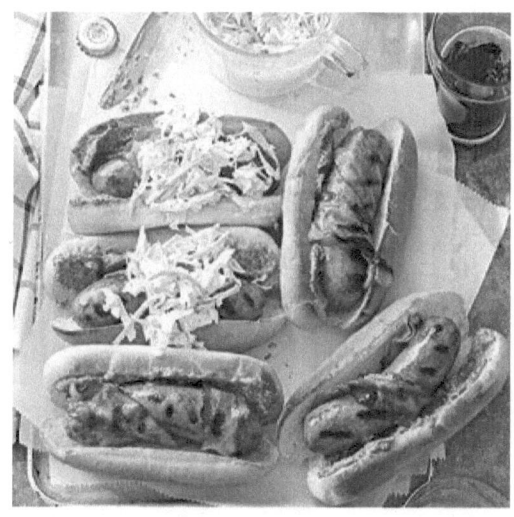

Ingredients

- 3 bratwurst links or turkey bratwursts, uncooked
- 6 ounces can German beer or ¾ cup beef broth
- 1 medium onion, chopped
- 1 ½ tablespoons bottled steak sauce
- 2 teaspoons smoked paprika
- 2 cloves garlic, chopped
- 3 slices bacon, uncooked
- 3 bratwurst buns or hot dog buns
- 2 ½ tablespoons coarsely ground mustard
- Tangy Midwest slaw to serve

Method

1. Using a fork, prick the skin of each bratwurst all over. In a large bowl, add beer, onion, steak sauce, paprika, garlic, and bratwurst. Mix well and transfer into a large Ziploc plastic bag. Place in the refrigerator for marinating for a minimum of 6 hours and a maximum of 24 hours. Turn the plastic bag a couple of times in between.

2. Transfer the entire contents of the bag into a saucepan. Place the saucepan over medium heat. Bring to a boil. Lower heat, cover and simmer for about 10 minutes. Meanwhile, place a skillet over medium heat. Add bacon and cook until browned. Remove with a slotted spoon and place on paper towels.

3. Remove the bratwurst from the saucepan and keep aside to cool. Discard the marinade. Place a bratwurst each over the bacon slices. Wrap the bratwurst with the bacon slices. Fasten it with wooden toothpicks. Grill the bratwurst in a preheated grill. When done, sprinkle mustard and serve with tangy Midwest slaw.

141. Texas Cowboy Style Ribs

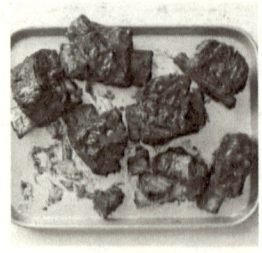

Ingredients

- 2 pounds beef chuck short ribs, trimmed of fat
- ½ tablespoon chili powder
- 1 ½ tablespoon packed brown sugar
- ½ teaspoon salt
- ½ teaspoon garlic powder
- 1 teaspoon onion powder
- ½ teaspoon ground cumin
- ½ teaspoon ground black pepper
- ¼ teaspoon cayenne pepper
- 1 cup mesquite wood chips
- 1 small onion, finely chopped
- 1 clove garlic, minced
- ½ tablespoon vegetable oil
- ¾ cup ketchup
- 2 tablespoons Worcestershire sauce
- 2 tablespoons hot, strong coffee
- 2 tablespoons red wine vinegar
- ½ can chipotle pepper in adobo sauce, chopped
- 1 teaspoon dry mustard
- ½ teaspoon salt or to taste

Method

1. Place the ribs in a baking dish. In a small bowl mix together chili powder, ½ tablespoon brown sugar, salt, garlic powder, onion powder, cumin, pepper and cayenne pepper. Sprinkle this mixture over the ribs all over. Rub with your hands.

2. Cover the dish with aluminum foil and bake in a preheated oven at 350-degree F for 1 ½ -2 hours or until done. Discard the fat. Soak the wood chips in water just enough to cover it, at least an hour before grilling. Drain the wood chips.

3. Place a saucepan over medium heat. Add oil. When heated, add onion and garlic and sauté until translucent. Add ketchup, Worcestershire sauce, coffee, vinegar, 1 tablespoon brown sugar, chipotle pepper, dry mustard, and salt. Bring to a boil. Lower heat; simmer for about 25-30 minutes.

4. Prepare a charcoal grill and sprinkle the wood chips over it. Place the grill rack directly over the coal. Place the ribs on the rack. Cover and

grill until the ribs are browned. Turn around the ribs a couple of times. Serve hot with the prepared sauce.

142. Grilled Corn with Chili and Manchego Cheese

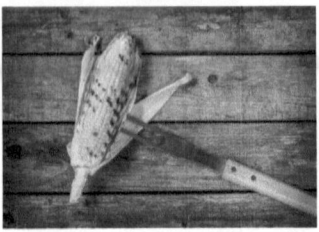

Ingredients

- 4-ounce Manchego cheese, finely grated
- ¾ cup butter at room temperature
- 2 small dried red chilies, finely chopped
- 2 tablespoons fresh flat leaf parsley, chopped
- Salt to taste
- Black pepper powder to taste
- A dozen ears of yellow corn with husk

Method

1. Mix together in a bowl, cheese, butter, chilli, salt, pepper, and parsley. Prepare a grill for medium heat. Lower the husks from the corn cobs and discard the corn silk. Pull the husks back around the corn. Place the corn on the grill. Cover and cook for around 15-20 minutes or until the corn is juicy and the husks are slightly blackish. Turn the corn cob a couple of times. Remove the husk from the corn and smear the cheese mixture over the hot corn and serve immediately.

143. Dressed Up Bacon Mac and Cheese

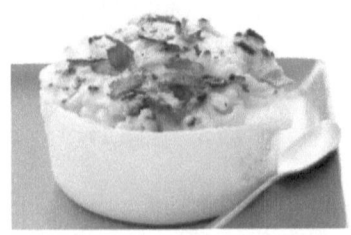

Ingredients

- 1 tablespoon unsalted butter
- 4 ounces macaroni, cooked according to instructions on the package, drained
- 1 ¼ cup cold milk
- 2-ounce provolone cheese, grated
- 42-ounce aged Asiago cheese, grated
- 1 large egg
- 1 scallion, white and green parts, chopped
- 2 slices white sandwich bread, torn into small pieces
- 2 strips bacon
- 1 small onion, chopped
- 1 clove garlic, minced
- 2 tablespoons all-purpose flour
- Cayenne pepper to taste
- Salt to taste

Method

1. Grease a casserole dish with unsalted butter. Add the macaroni and 2 tablespoons cold milk. In a small bowl, beat egg with 2 tablespoons of milk. In another bowl, mix together both the cheeses. Add half the cheese to the egg mixture along with scallion, and bread.

2. Place a skillet over medium heat. Add the bacon and cook until crisp. Remove with a slotted spoon and place over paper towels. When cool, crumble the bacon. Retain only about a tablespoon of the fat remaining in the skillet and discard the rest. Add onions and garlic and sauté until the onions are browned. Add flour, cayenne pepper, and salt. Sauté for a couple of minutes. Add the remaining milk and about ½ cup water gradually. Stir constantly until it thickens. Bring to a boil and remove from heat.

3. Cool for about 5-7 minutes and add the remaining cheese. Combine the sauce and macaroni. Add the bacon to the bread mixture. Transfer the bread mixture over the pasta. Spread evenly all over. Place the casserole dish in a preheated oven at 375-degree F for about 40 minutes. Remove from oven and cool for about 10 minutes before serving.

144. Garlicky Summer Squash and Fresh Corn

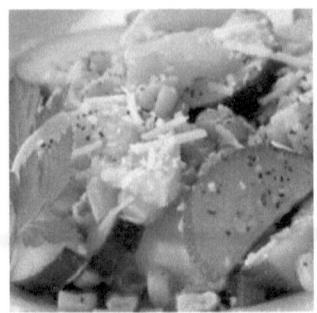

Ingredients

- ¼ cup olive oil
- 1 yellow onion, sliced
- 10 cloves garlic, minced
- 1 cup vegetable broth
- 2 ears corn, remove kernels cut from cob
- 4 cups yellow squash, sliced
- 4 cups zucchini, sliced
- 2 tablespoons fresh parsley, chopped
- ¼ cup butter
- Salt to taste
- Pepper powder to taste

Method

1. Place a skillet over medium heat. Add oil. When the oil is heated up, add onions and garlic. Sauté until the onions are translucent. Add vegetable broth and corn kernels. Bring to a boil.

2. Add zucchini and squash. Stir, cover, and cook for about 10-15 minutes until the vegetables are tender. Add salt, pepper, parsley, and butter. Cook until the butter melts. Serve immediately.

145. Daddy's Fried Corn and Onion

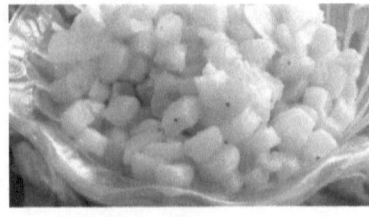

Ingredients

- 2 ears fresh corn, remove the kernels
- 1 tablespoon butter
- 1 small sweet onion, diced
- Salt to taste
- Pepper powder to taste

Method

1. Place a skillet over medium heat. Add corn kernels and sauté for a few minutes until the corn is tender. Add onions and sauté until the onions are just about to turn crisp. Add salt and pepper, mix well, and serve. Can be served either warm or cold.

146. Baked 3-Bean Casserole

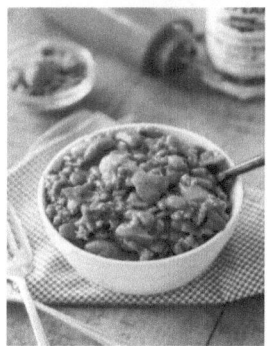

Ingredients

- ½ a 16 ounce can maple cured bacon baked beans
- ½ a 16 ounce can hot chili beans, undrained
- ½ a 15 ounce can black beans, rinsed, drained
- ½ a 10 ounce can diced tomatoes and green chilies, undrained
- 1 teaspoon minced chipotle peppers in adobo sauce

Method

1. Mix together all the ingredients in a greased baking dish. Cover with a foil. Bake in a preheated oven at 350-degree F for about an hour. Remove the foil and bake for 15 minutes. Serve hot.

147. Grilled Mussels

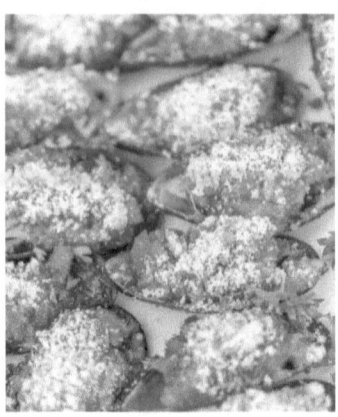

Summary

Enjoy this delicious summer dinner with a chilled glass of dry white wine.

Ingredients

- 1 lbs. Mussels
- 1 (14.5oz.) can Diced Tomatoes
- ¼ cup White Wine
- 2 tbsps. Olive Oil
- 2 cloves Garlic (minced)
- 1 tsp Crushed Red Pepper Flakes
- 1 Bay Leaf

Method

1. Place a large skill on the grill over medium heat. Add olive oil, pepper flakes, and garlic. Cook 1 minute, stirring constantly. Add wine, tomatoes, and bay leaf. Simmer 5 minutes. Add mussels. Cover. Cook 8 minutes.

Health Benefits of Mussels

High in Omega 3 Fatty Acids. High in Zinc, Iron, and Folic Acid. 1 cup of mussels contains 30% of daily protein.

148. Gazpacho

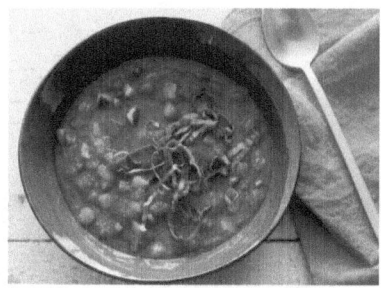

Summary

This gazpacho is the best way to cool off when you're in the mood for something more savory.

Ingredients

- 2 ¼ lbs. Tomatoes (cut in wedges)
- 3 oz. Bell Peppers (chopped)
- 2 oz. Cucumber (chopped
- 2 Onions (cut in wedges)
- 3 cloves Garlic (halved)
- 1 ¼ oz. Country Style Bread (crust removed, torn)
- ½ cup water
- 1/3 cup Olive Oil
- 2 Tbsps. Sherry Vinegar
- 1 Tbsp. Mayonnaise
- 4 oz. Croutons

Method

1. Fill a small pan with cold water and garlic. Bring to a boil. Once boiling, remove garlic. Transfer to a bowl of ice water. In a bowl, combine tomatoes, onions, garlic, cucumbers, bell peppers, and bread. Toss to combine. Add water. Blend until smooth with a stick blender.

2. Add mayonnaise, vinegar, and oil. Whisk until thoroughly blended. Season with salt and pepper. Chill 2 hours. Serve topped with croutons and a drizzle of oil.

Raw Power

This raw recipe allows you to preserve certain nutrients which are otherwise destroyed in cooking. Vitamin C is one of the most sensitive to heat so you need to eat veggies raw to make sure you get enough. B vitamins are also destroyed by heat.

149. Tuna & Eggplant Salad in a Jar

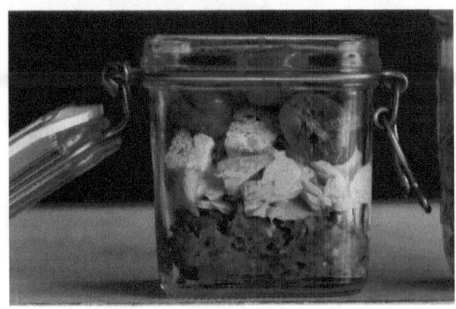

Summary

Make these hearty and delicious salads in bulk and take them with you when you go to work or out for a hike.

Ingredients

- 2 (6oz.) cans Tuna Packed in Olive Oil
- 1 large Anchovy Fillet
- ¼ cup Mayonnaise
- 2 (13oz.) jars Grilled Eggplant
- 2 cups Breadcrumbs
- 2 cups Grape Tomatoes (halved)
- 1/3 cup Fresh Mint (chopped)
- 1/3 cup Fresh Basil (chopped)
- 2 Tbsps. Olive Oil
- 2 tsp Fresh Lemon Juice
- 2 tsp Drained Capers
- 1 tsp Garlic (chopped)
- 1 tsp Lemon Zest
- 1 tsp Red Wine Vinegar

Method

1. In a blender, combine lemon juice, oil, mayonnaise, capers, anchovy, and ¼ cup tuna. Blend until smooth. In a food processor, pulse together garlic, eggplant, zest, parsley, and vinegar until combined.

2. In a bowl, toss together tomatoes and mint. Divide eggplant mixture into sanitized jars. Layer in remaining tuna. Add sauce from the blender. Top with tomatoes. Drizzle olive oil over the top.

Fishy Nutrients

Oily fish like tuna and anchovy have some of the highest amounts of Omega-3s. Omega-3 protects your brain and heart from damage caused by age, pollution, or smoke. The unsaturated fats in the fish helps your body better absorb the vitamins from the veggies in this recipe.

150. Peanut Butter & Berry Pie

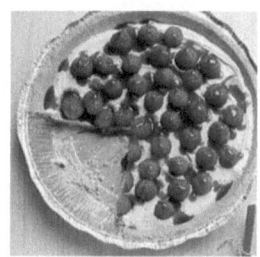

Summary

Forget PB&Js. Try this pie version of the American classic instead.

Ingredients

- 1 Oat Pie Crust
- 4 Eggs
- 1 ¼ cup Evaporated Milk
- ½ cup Peanut Butter
- 1 cup Mini Marshmallows
- 1-pint Fresh Raspberries
- 1 tsp Vanilla Extract
- 2 Tbsps. Raspberry Jam (warmed)

Method

1. Preheat oven to 350°F. Chill crust 15 minutes. Remove from fridge. Lightly prick the crust all over with a fork. Line with parchment paper. Fill with uncooked rice (or pie weights). Bake 30 minutes. Let cool.

2. Remove parchment paper with rice. Increase oven temperature to 400°F. Spread jam across bottom of crust. In a bowl, whisk together vanilla extract and eggs. Heat milk, peanut butter, and sugar in a pot over medium heat until steaming. Whisk constantly. Whisk milk mixture into egg mixture until combined. Spoon into pie crust. Bake 15 minutes. Top with marshmallows. Bake additional 1-2 minutes. Let cool 3 hours. Top with raspberries. Serve.

Sugar-Free Tips

Replace marshmallows with honey-sweetened whipped cream. Find or make your own raspberry jam with natural sugar substitutes (like stevia). Make your own natural, healthier peanut butter by simply grinding peanuts in a food processor until it becomes creamy.

151. Plum Semifreddo

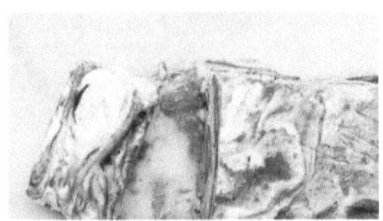

Summary

This frozen custard-like dish is a welcome sight on a hot day.

Ingredients

- 1 ½ lbs. Red Plums (cut in chunks)
- 1 cup Chilled Heavy Cream
- 1 cup Sugar
- 3 large Egg Whites
- ½ tsp Ground Cardamom
- ½ tsp Vanilla Extract
- Olive Oil
- Salt

Method

1. Grease a (9"x5") baking dish. Line with plastic wrap (should hang over the sides. In a pan over medium heat, mix plums, 1/3 cup sugar,

cardamom, and salt. Cover. Cook 5 minutes, stirring occasionally. Uncover. Cook an additional 6-8 minutes. Let cool 5 minutes. Puree mixture in a blender until smooth. Strain through fine sieve into a bowl. Press on solids to release juice. Set aside 1 cup of puree. Let cool.

2. In a heatproof bowl, whisk together egg whites, 2/3 cup sugar, and a dash of salt. Set bowl over a saucepan filled with simmering water (without letting bowl touch water) for 4 minutes. Remove from heat. Add vanilla. Beat vigorously (or with mixer) until glossy and tripled in volume. Let cool.

3. In another bowl, whip cream into soft peaks. Mix whipped cream into egg white mixture in 1/3 cup batches. Fold in plum puree. Combine until streaks of puree appear throughout mixture (do not blend completely). Pour mixture into prepared baking dish. Smooth surface. Fold plastic wrap over the top. Freeze 8 hours. Drizzle reserved cup of puree over top before serving.

Health Benefits of Plums

A single plum contains 113mg of potassium which you need to regulate blood pressure and decrease risk of stroke. Plums are high in fiber. Eating plums daily strengthens bones.

152. Cherry Bourbon Ice Cream

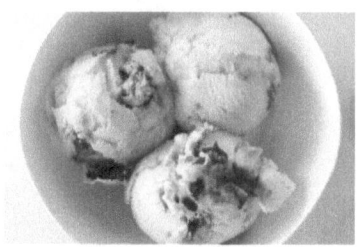

Summary

Cool down with this spiked ice cream recipe.

Ingredients

- 1 ½ cups Dark Cherries (pitted, halved)
- 2 Tbsps. Sugar
- 1 Tbsp. Water

- 1 Tbsp. Bourbon
- 1 ½ cups Heavy Cream
- 1 cup Whole Milk
- ½ cup Sugar
- 5 Egg Yolks
- 1 tsp Vanilla Extract
- 1 pinch Salt

Method

1. In a small pan on medium heat, combine cherries, 1 tablespoon sugar, and water. Cook 8-10 minutes, stirring occasionally. Remove from heat. Stir in bourbon. Let cool.

2. Whisk together heavy cream, milk, egg yolks, ½ cup sugar, and pinch of salt until fluffy. Fold cherry mixture into custard. Do not over mix. Let streaks of cherry mixture remain. Chill in freezer 3 hours.

Health Benefits of Cherries

High in antioxidants that help prevent cancer. Helps treat pain from arthritis or gout. High in melatonin that helps you sleep better.

153. Open Faced Eggplant & Basil Sandwiches

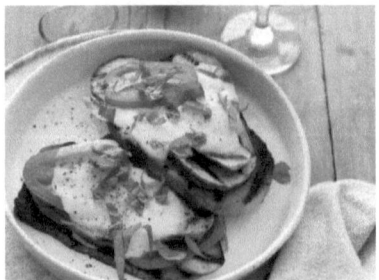

Summary

Pack these simple sandwiches for lunch or a picnic this summer.

Ingredients

- 1 lbs. Eggplant (cubed)
- 8 slices Country Style Bread
- ½ cup Fresh Basil Leaves (torn)

- 1 oz. Parmesan (shaved)
- 1 Tbsp. Fresh Lemon Juice
- 8 Tbsps. Olive Oil
- 2cloves Garlic (sliced)
- 1 tsp Oregano (or Marjoram)
- ¼ tsp Crushed Red Pepper Flakes
- Salt & Pepper to taste

Method

1. Heat 4 tablespoons oil in large pan on medium heat. Add oregano, pepper flakes, and garlic. Cook 2 minutes, stirring often. Add eggplant. Cook 8-10 minutes, tossing occasionally.

2. Add ½ cup water. Season with salt and pepper. Cook 10-15 minutes, tossing occasionally. Let cool 5 minutes. Stir in lemon juice. Prepare grill for medium-high heat. Brush both sides of bread slices generously with oil. Grill 1-2 minutes each side. Spoon eggplant mixture onto toast. Top with parmesan and basil.

Health Benefits of Eggplant

Contain phytonutrients that improve circulation and strengthen the brain. High in fiber which prevents colon cancer and help manage diabetes. Contain bioflavonoids which prevent blood clots and strengthen capillaries.

154. Corn Zucchini Feta Salad

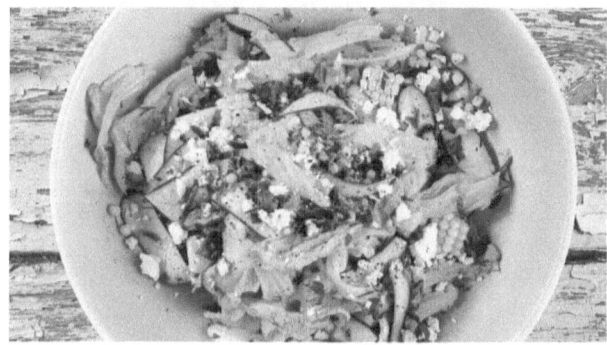

Summary

This quick salad is delicious and satisfying.

Ingredients

- 4 ears Corn
- 4 small Zucchini (thinly sliced lengthwise)
- 8-10 Zucchini Blossoms (torn)
- ¼ cup Fresh Basil (chopped)
- ¼ cup Fresh Parsley (chopped)
- 1/3 cup Olive Oil
- ¼ cup White Wine Vinegar
- 1 cup Feta (crumbled)
- ½ tsp Crushed Red Pepper Flakes
- Salt & Pepper to Taste

Method

1. Boil corn 3 minutes. Remove from water. Let cool on plate. Cut kernels away from cob into a large bowl. Add zucchini, parsley, basil, pepper flakes, oil and vinegar. Toss to combine. Season with salt and pepper. Top with feta crumbles. Serve.

Health Benefits of Zucchini

High in heart-protecting potassium. When shredded, they make an extra healthy substitute for pasta noodles! High in cholesterol-fighting minerals.

155. Buttery Salmon with Hazelnut Relish

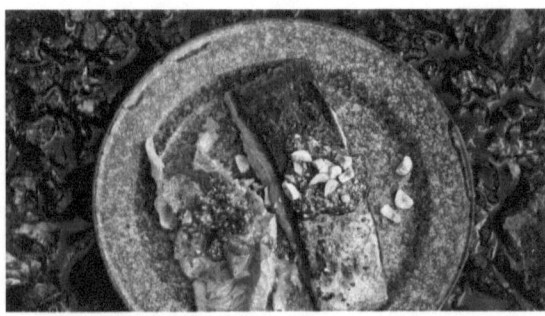

Summary

Lighten up your dinner without sacrificing flavor and satisfaction with this recipe.

Ingredients

- 2 small heads Lettuce
- 1 cup Fresh Cilantro
- ½ cup Fresh Parsley
- 4 (6oz.) Salmon Fillets (with skin)
- ½ cup Blanched Hazelnuts
- ½ cup Olive Oil
- 2 Tbsps. Butter
- 1 Tbsp. Olive Oil
- 1 Tbsp. Capers
- 1 clove Garlic (chopped)
- 1 tsp Lemon Zest
- Salt to taste

Method

1. Preheat oven to 400°F. Arrange hazelnuts on rimmed baking sheet. Bake 6-8 minutes, tossing occasionally. Let cool. In a processor, pulse together parsley, cilantro, garlic, lemon zest, capers, and ¼ cup hazelnuts. Gradually add olive oil while still pulsing. Season with salt. Transfer to bowl. Add remaining hazelnuts to processor. Chop coarsely. Heat oil in a large (ovenproof) pan on medium-high heat.

2. Lightly salt salmon. Cook skin side down 4 minutes. Add butter to pan. Cook 1-minute, basting salmon constantly. Transfer pan to oven. Roast 3 minutes, basting once. Serve salmon skin side up. Top with lettuce, cilantro mixture and chopped hazelnuts.

Health Benefits of Hazelnuts

High in muscle-building magnesium. 1 cup of hazelnuts contains more than 80% of your daily Vitamin E (which maintains your skin's youthful glow). High in energizing and rejuvenating B vitamins.

156. Steak Okra Tomato Kebabs

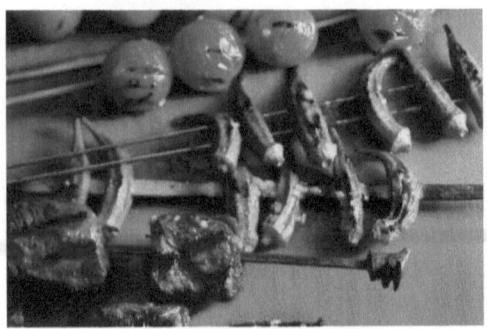

Summary

These quick kebabs are perfect for spontaneous backyard parties.

Ingredients

- ¾ lbs. Okra
- 1 lbs. Small Tomatoes
- 2 lbs. Boneless Chuck Blade Steak (trimmed, cubed)
- ½ cup Olive Oil
- 3 Tbsps. Shallot (chopped)
- 3 Tbsps. Red Wine Vinegar
- 2 tsp Dijon Mustard
- ½ tsp Sugar
- 16 metal skewers

Method

1. In a bowl, blend mustard, vinegar, shallots, sugar, salt and pepper. Slowly drizzle in oil, whisking constantly. Rub steak with ½ teaspoon salt. Place in Ziploc bag with 6 tablespoons oil-vinegar mixture. Toss to coat. Marinate 2 hours. Chill remaining oil-vinegar mixture. Prepare grill for medium-high heat.

2. In a bowl, toss okra and tomatoes with 3 tablespoons oil and ¼ teaspoon salt. Place all the tomatoes onto skewers (lining up full skewers with just tomatoes). Pierce a skewer through each end of 1 okra. Add the remaining okra pierces onto the pair of skewers. Set aside. Chop steak into pieces. Places pieces onto skewers. Grill steak skewers 5 minutes, turning once. Transfer to platter. Drizzle with some oil-vinegar mixture. Grill okra and tomato skewers 8 minutes. Transfer to steak platter. Serve with remaining oil-vinegar mixture.

Health Benefits of Okra

Helps stabilize blood sugar. May help prevent asthma attacks. Reduces acne outbreaks.

157. Pork Chops Topped with Pickled Watermelon Salad

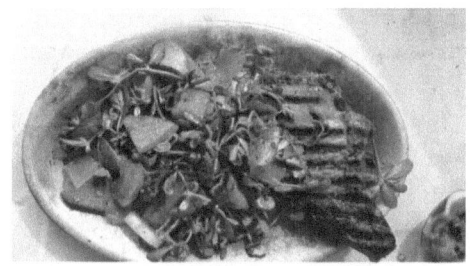

Summary

Pickled watermelon salad puts a unique twist on this pork chop dinner.

Ingredients

- 4 Bone-In Pork Chops
- 2 Shallots (sliced into rings)
- ¼ cup Low Sodium Soy Sauce
- 2 Tbsps. Fish Sauce
- 2 Tbsps. Sugar
- 1 tsp Sriracha Sauce
- ½ cup Pickled Watermelon Rind (sliced)
- ½ lbs. Watermelon Flesh (seeded, cubed)
- 4 cups Arugula
- 4 Shallots (sliced)
- 6 Tbsps. Olive Oil
- 1 Tbsp. Rice Vinegar
- 1 tsp Low Sodium Soy Sauce
- ¼ tsp Sugar
- Salt & Pepper to taste

Method

1. In a baking dish, blend together fish sauce, soy sauce, Sriracha, sugar, and shallots. Add pork chops. Turn to coat. Cover. Chill 1 hour,

turning occasionally. Heat 4 tablespoons oil in a small pan on medium heat.

2. Add shallots (from pork marinade) to pan. Cook 4 minutes. Drain on paper towels. In a bowl, whisk together remaining oil with soy sauce, vinegar, and sugar. Season with salt and pepper. Add watermelon and pickled watermelon rind. Toss to coat. Prepare grill for medium-high heat. Remove pork chops from marinade. Grill 3 minutes per side. Top with fried shallots. Serve with watermelon salad.

Health Benefits of Watermelon Rinds

Contains immune system-boosting citrulline. Eaten before a workout, can help prevent muscle fatigue and improve endurance. May help with erectile dysfunction.

158. Porterhouse Steak with Herbed Butter

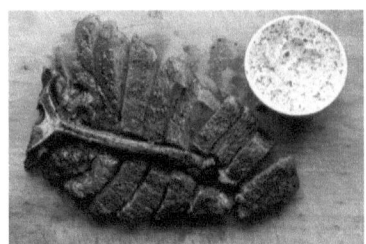

Summary

This simple dish embraces the natural flavors of each ingredient.

Ingredients

- 2 Porterhouse Steaks
- 2 Tbsps. Olive Oil
- 2 Tbsps. Butter
- ¼ cup Mixed Fresh Herbs (your preference)
- ½ cup Butter
- Salt & Pepper to taste

Method

1. Let steak sit out at room temperature 30 minutes. In a bowl, stir together butter and herbs with wooden spoon. Season with salt and

pepper. Cover with plastic wrap. Chill at least 1 hour. Preheat oven to 350°F. Pat steaks dry. Season with salt and pepper.

2. Heat 1 tablespoon oil in pan on medium-heat. When oil smokes, add steak. Cook 3 minutes per side. Melt 1 tablespoon butter in pan. Spoon over steak. Remove from pan. Set aside. Repeat for second steak. Place steaks on rimmed baking sheet with a wire rack. Bake until meat thermometer reads 120°-125°F. Transfer to wooden board. Let rest 10 minutes. Serve with herbed butter.

Health Benefits of Fresh Herbs

Fresh rosemary improves concentration and memory. Fresh parsley helps prevent breast cancer. Fresh mint relives symptoms of irritable bowel syndrome.

159. Grilled Panzanella

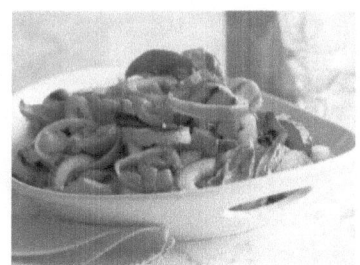

Summary

This hearty grilled salad can hold its own at any barbecue.

Ingredients

- 1 lbs. Cherry Tomatoes (grilled)
- 1 bunch Scallions
- 1 clove Garlic (halved)
- 2 cups Arugula
- 2 Tbsps. Olive Oil
- 2 Tbsps. Red Wine Vinegar
- Salt & Pepper to taste
- 4 thick slices Country Style Bread (crust removed)

Method

1. In a bowl, toss together scallions, oil, salt and pepper. Grill on high heat 4 minutes, turning occasionally. Let cool. Chop. Brush both sides of each bread slice generously with oil. Grill bread on high heat 2 minutes each side. Rub all sides vigorously with garlic. Tear into pieces. Toss together with tomatoes, scallions, Arugula, oil, and vinegar.

Health Benefits of Tomatoes

Tomatoes are high in cancer-fighting lycopene (which your body absorbs more easily from cooked tomatoes). Lycopene helps protect your skin from sun damage. The vitamin A in tomatoes protects your eyes from macular degeneration.

160. Zucchini Patties

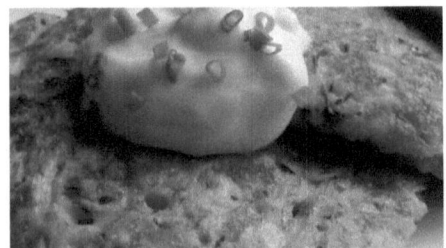

Summary

These patties are the best way to sneak a serving of veggies onto your dinner plate.

Ingredients

- 4 medium Zucchini (grated)
- 1 Onion (grated)
- 1 leek (chopped)
- 2 large Eggs (beaten)
- 1/3 cup Breadcrumbs
- 1 ½ cups Vegetable Oil
- 1 Tbsp. Thyme
- Salt & Pepper to taste
- Roasted Red Pepper Labneh

Method

1. In a bowl, combine zucchini, onion, and 3 teaspoons salt. Toss to coat. Let sit 10 minutes. Place zucchini mixture in a paper towel and squeeze to wring out juice.

2. Transfer to a new bowl. Add leek, breadcrumbs, egg, and thyme. Season with pepper. Heat oil in a deep pan on medium heat. Drop spoonful of zucchini mix into hot oil. Gently flatten with spoon. Cook 3 minutes per side. Drain on paper towels. Serve with labneh.

More Health Benefits of Zucchini

High fiber content helps control appetite and improve digestion. The fiber also helps sweep toxins out of your body. B vitamins, zinc, and magnesium help your body break down blood sugars.

161. Chicken Salad with Crème Fraiche and Rye

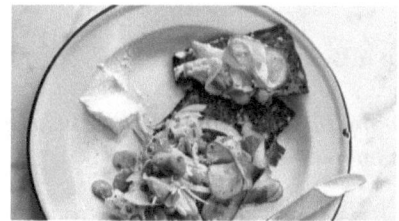

Summary

This chicken salad is beautifully accented with crème fraiche and summery flavors.

Ingredients

- 12-14 oz. Bone-In Chicken Breast
- 4 Tbsps. Olive Oil
- ¾ cup Fava Beans (fresh)
- ½ bulb Fennel (sliced)
- 1 Scallion (sliced)
- ½ cup Crème Fraiche
- ½ Cucumber (thinly sliced lengthwise)
- ¼ cup Fresh Parsley
- 1 Tbsp. Sherry Vinegar
- 2 Tbsps. Fresh Tarragon (chopped)

- ½ tsp Lemon Zest
- 2 tsp Fresh Lemon Juice
- 8 slices Rye Bread
- Salt & Pepper to taste

Method

1. Preheat oven to 425°F. Arrange chicken on a rimmed baking sheet. Rub with 1 tablespoon oil, salt, and pepper. Roast 25-30 minutes. Let cool. Shred into bite-sized chunks. Boil fava beans 4 minutes. Drain. Transfer to bowl of ice water. In a large bowl, toss together fava beans, fennel, chicken, scallions, tarragon, oil, vinegar, salt and pepper. In a separate bowl, whisk crème fraiche to soft peaks (fluffy). Sprinkle in salt.

2. In a third bowl, toss together cucumber, parsley, lemon zest, and lemon juice. Season with salt and pepper. Divide chicken salad and cucumber mixture into bowls. Add a dollop of crème fraiche. Serve with bread.

Health Benefits of Fava Beans

High in bone-strengthening phosphorous. High in heart-protecting magnesium and potassium. High in immune-boosting folate.

162. Lobster Spaghetti

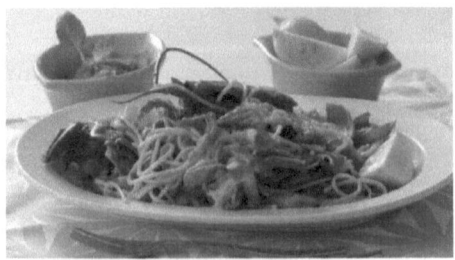

Summary

Upgrade your spaghetti dinner with lobster.

Ingredients

- 12 oz. Spaghetti
- 1 lbs. Lobster Meat (cooked)

- 1 lbs. Cherry Tomatoes (halved)
- 1 Shallot (chopped)
- 2 Tbsps. Olive Oil
- 2 Tbsps. Butter
- 1 tsp Lemon Zest
- 1 tsp. Crushed Red Pepper Flakes
- Salt & Pepper to taste

Method

1. Cook spaghetti until al dente. Drain. Reserve 1 cup liquid. Heat oil and butter in a large pan on medium-high heat. Add shallot and pepper flakes. Cook 2 minutes, stirring often.

2. Add tomatoes. Cook 5-8 minutes, stirring often. Add lobster meat. Toss to coat. Add pasta plus ½ cup reserved liquid. Season with salt and pepper. Cook 2 minutes, tossing constantly. Add more liquid as needed to thicken sauce and evenly coat pasta. Divide onto plates. Garnish with lemon zest and wedges.

Health Benefits of Lobster

Naturally low in cholesterol and high in protein. High in thyroid-boosting selenium which helps control weight. Helps lower blood pressure.

163. Melon Soup

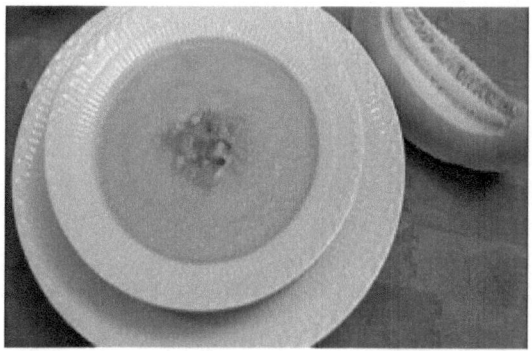

Summary

Melons turn this soup into a refreshing and smooth meal.

Ingredients

- 4 oz. Silken Tofu
- ¼ cup White Soy Sauce
- 6 lbs. Melons (very ripe)
- ¼ cup Almond Oil
- ¼ cup Toasted Almonds
- 1 Onion (sliced)
- 10 Tbsps. Butter
- Sherry Vinegar
- Fresh Herb Blend (your preference)
- Salt to taste

Method

1. Press tofu through a fine sieve into a bowl. Stir in soy sauce. Cover and chill. Scoop out 18 melon balls into a bowl. Season with salt and vinegar. Toss gently. Let stand 30 minutes. Drain. Transfer to a new bowl. Set aside. Cut rind from remaining melon. Chop flesh into 2" cubes. Melt 6 tablespoons butter in a large pot on medium-low heat. Add onion. Cook 10 minutes, stirring often. Cut out a piece of parchment paper large enough to cover the opening of the pot.

2. Add melon cubes to pot along with remaining butter. Cover with parchment paper. Simmer 15 minutes, stirring occasionally. Remove from heat. Let cool 5 minutes. Puree soup into blender until smooth. Cover and chill 4 hours. Ladle soup into chilled bowls. Dollop tofu mixture on top. Garnish with toasted almonds, fresh herbs, and melon balls. Drizzle with almond oil.

Health Benefits of Melons

High in Vitamin A which is good for skin, hair, teeth, nails and eyes. Helps improve metabolism. Acts as a natural anti-inflammatory.

164. Pan-Fried Shishito Peppers

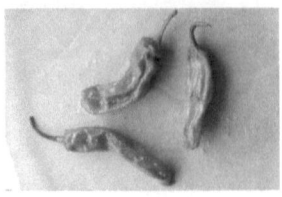

Summary

This elegantly simple side dish will pair perfectly with steak, pork, poultry, or fish.

Ingredients

- Shishito Peppers
- Olive Oil
- Fresh Lemon Juice
- Salt

Method

1. Heat oil in a large pan on medium heat. Add peppers. Cook 10-15 minutes, tossing frequently. Remove from heat. Sprinkle in salt. Drizzle in lemon. Toss to coat.

Health Benefits of Shishito Peppers

High in cancer-fighting antioxidants. Boost immune system function. Act as natural anti-inflammatory.

165. Sweet & Savory Summer Salad

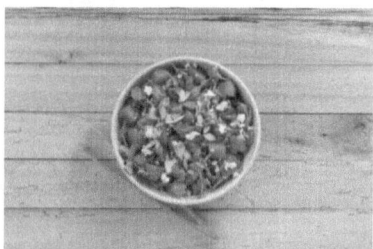

Summary

This salad combines the perfect balance of hearty protein and fruity notes.

Ingredients

- 10 large Eggs
- 1/3 cup Flour
- 1 cup Lemon Vinaigrette
- 1-quart Vegetable Oil

- ¾ cup Raw Shelled Pistachios
- 8 small Apricots (pitted, diced)
- 1 ¼ cup Mixed Fresh Herbs (your preference)
- 4 cups Arugula
- 2/3 cup Blanched Whole Almonds (ground)
- 2/3 cup Parmesan (grated)
- 1 cup Breadcrumbs
- Salt & Pepper to taste

Method

1. Prepare a large bowl with ice water. Set aside. Bring water to a boil. Add 8 eggs. Reduce heat. Simmer 6 minutes. Transfer eggs to ice water. Let stand 5 minutes. Peel. Set aside. In a bowl, whisk together flour, salt, and pepper. In another bowl, beat together 2 eggs with 2 tablespoons water. In a third bowl, blend breadcrumbs, ground almonds, parmesan, salt and pepper. Roll boiled eggs in flour mixture one at a time. Dip into breadcrumb mixture and then egg mixture. Repeat steps. Place coated eggs on baking sheet and chill in fridge 30 minutes.

2. In a large bowl, toss together ½ cup pistachios, ½ cup apricots, herbs, and arugula. Heat 3" oil in a large pan on high heat. Carefully fry eggs 1-2 minutes per side. Drain on paper towels. Drizzle vinaigrette over salad. Toss to coat. Divide salad into 8 bowls. Garnish with remaining pistachios and apricots and 1 egg (sliced).

Health Benefits of Arugula

High in brain-boosting folate. High in fiber which controls appetite, improves digestion, and detoxes the body. High in bone-strengthening Vitamin K.

166. Summery Spinach

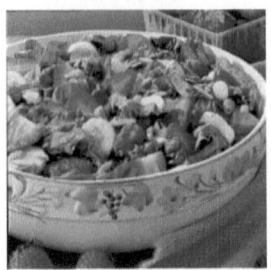

Summary

Spinach is the star of this simple side dish.

Ingredients

- 4 large bunches Fresh Spinach
- 2 cloves Garlic (halved)
- Olive Oil
- ½ Lemon
- Salt to taste

Method

1. Heat oil in a large pot over medium-high heat. Add garlic. Stir 1 minute. Remove garlic. Add spinach. Salt to taste. Cut leaves with scissors as they wilt. Once wilted, arrange spinach on a platter. Drizzle lemon juice over.

Health Benefits of Spinach

Cooking spinach removes the oxalic acid which prevents your body from absorbing the high calcium and iron contents found in the leaves. A diet with lots of spinach helps relieve itchy or dry skin. Spinach helps treat constipation and prevent ulcers.

167. Avocado Plum Salad

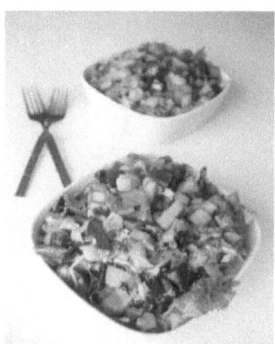

Summary

Avocado and plum bring the best of both worlds into this salad.

Ingredients

- 2 Ripe Hass Avocados (pitted, peeled, chopped)
- 5 Ripe Black Plums (pitted, chopped)
- 1 cup Fresh Cilantro (chopped)
- 1 Lemon
- 1 Red Chili Pepper (dried, chopped)
- 1 clove Garlic (minced)
- ½ cup Olive Oil
- Salt to taste

Method

1. In a bowl, carefully combine plum and avocado. Do not mix too much (or avocado will get mushy). Squeeze lemon juice over and sprinkle with salt. Smash garlic together with salt to form a paste. Add chili pepper. Continue to crush. Add cilantro. Continue crushing. Whisk in olive oil. Drizzle dressing over the plum and avocado.

Health Benefits of Avocados

High in unsaturated fats that help control appetite, hydrate skin, and absorb nutrients. Avocados contain more potassium than bananas. Help lower cholesterol.

168. Summer Picnic Rolls

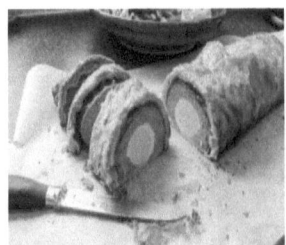

Summary

These simple little treats are the perfect dish to pack for a picnic.

Ingredients

- 1 oz. Cellophane Noodles
- 1 lbs. Ground Turkey Breast (extra lean)

- 2 large Egg Whites (beaten)
- 1 cup Scallions (chopped)
- ½ cup Shiitake Mushrooms (chopped)
- 1 cup Canned Mung Bean Sprouts (drained)
- 9 (8") sheets Rice Paper
- ½ Red Bell Pepper (thinly sliced)
- ½ Green Bell Pepper (thinly sliced)
- 2 tsp Olive Oil
- 1 tsp Sugar
- 1 tsp Fish Sauce
- 1 tsp Oyster Sauce
- ¼ tsp Pepper

Method

1. Boil noodles for 3 minutes. Drain. Set aside. In a bowl, mix together turkey, fish sauce, egg whites, oyster sauce, mushrooms, scallions, sugar, and pepper.

2. Heat oil in a large pan on medium-high heat. Cook turkey mixture 7 minutes, stir to crumble. Remove from heat. Push turkey to one side. Add pepper to other side. Soak rice paper in a bowl of warm water 10-15 seconds for each piece. Lay flat. Evenly distribute all ingredients onto each paper. Fold bottom edge up. Fold in the sides. Roll up toward the top edge.

Health Benefits of Mung Bean Sprouts

High in fiber. High in vitamin C. High in vitamin K.

169. Sweet Corn Soup

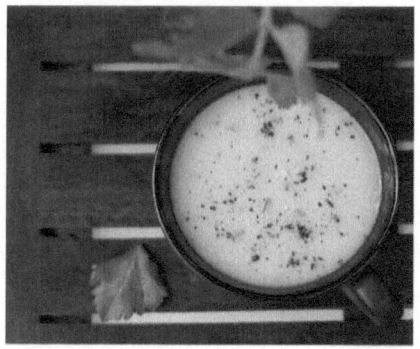

Summary

This sweet corn soup can stand alone or be paired with fresh fish tacos.

Ingredients

- 2 quarts Vegetable Stock
- 6 ears Sweet Corn
- 2 large Onions (diced)
- 4 large stalks Celery (sliced)
- 1 ½ lbs. Potatoes (diced)
- 1 ½ cups Whole Milk
- ½ cup Fresh Parsley (chopped)
- 3 Tbsps. Olive Oil
- 1 tsp Cayenne Pepper
- 1 tsp Ground Coriander
- ½ tsp Paprika
- Salt & Pepper to taste

Method

1. In a large pot, bring stock to a boil. Reduce heat. Let simmer. Place the corn cobs in the pot. Simmer 20 minutes. Heat oil in a large pan over medium heat. Add onions. Cook 3 minutes. Add thyme and celery. Cook 4 minutes. Turn off heat. Remove corn cobs from stock. Add cooked veggies, potatoes, paprika, cayenne, coriander, salt, and pepper. Simmer 25 minutes. Scrape kernels from cobs. Stir in corn kernels and milk. Simmer 3 minutes. Puree 1 quart of soup in a blender until smooth.

2. Return pureed soup to pot. Let simmer, stirring frequently. Hold the bell pepper with tongs over an open flame on the stove. Turn frequently to char all sides. Remove skin, stem, and seeds. Dice bell pepper. Remove soup from heat. Stir in parsley, salt, and pepper. Ladle into bowls and garnish with bell pepper.

Busting Corn Myths

Corn is full of healthy nutrients and contains less sugar than an apple. Corn is actually healthier when cooked as more antioxidants get released. Corn is high in fiber.

170. Summer Slaw

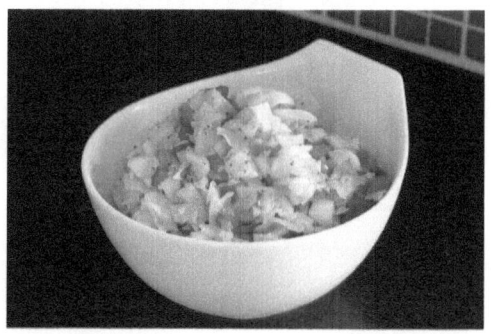

Summary

Broccoli turns normal slaw into a deliciously summer experience.

Ingredients

- 2/3 cup Buttermilk
- 1/3 cup Mayonnaise
- 1 small head Broccoli
- ½ head Cabbage (thinly sliced)
- ½ lbs. Sugar Snap Peas (sliced)
- 4 Tbsps. Chives (chopped)
- 3 Tbsps. Fresh Lemon Juice
- 2 Scallions (sliced)
- Salt & Pepper to taste

Method

1. In a bowl, whisk together buttermilk, lemon juice, mayonnaise, salt and pepper. Set aside. Halve broccoli pieces lengthwise. Thinly slice crosswise. In a large bowl, toss together broccoli, peas, scallions, cabbage, 2 tablespoons chives, and buttermilk dressing. Season with salt and pepper. Garnish with remaining chives.

Health Benefits of Broccoli

Helps lower cholesterol. Helps treat symptoms of allergies. Just ½ a cup of broccoli per day can dramatically lower your risk for cancer.

171. Marinated Summer Veggies

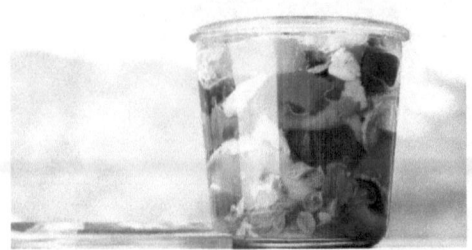

Summary

This recipe makes the absolute perfect side dish to a steak or pork chop.

Ingredients

- 1 lbs. Summer Squash or Zucchini (sliced diagonally)
- 3 Red Bell Peppers (sliced)
- 2 cloves Garlic
- 5 Tbsps. Olive Oil
- 2 Tbsps. Red Wine Vinegar
- 4 sprigs Oregano
- Salt & Pepper to taste

Method

1. Preheat oven to 475°F. Place squash and peppers each on their own baking sheets. Drizzle 1 tablespoon oil over each. Season with salt and pepper. Toss to coat. Spread out in a single layer.

2. Roast peppers on higher rack in oven. Roast squash on lower rack. Cook 15-20 minutes. Remove skins from peppers. In a bowl, whisk together vinegar, 3 tablespoons oil, garlic, salt and pepper. Add roasted vegetables and oregano. Toss to coat. Cover and let sit 1 hour. Serve.

Health Benefits of Bell Peppers

Amazingly high in vitamin A. High in capsaicin which help with weight loss and diabetes. High in lutein and other eye-protecting nutrients.

172. Pan-Fried Summer Squash

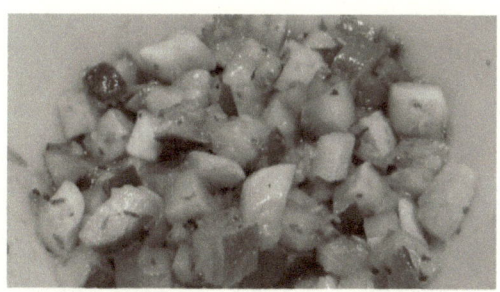

Summary

Squash and almonds come together in perfect harmony in this exquisite dish.

Ingredients

- 2 lbs. Summer Squash or Zucchini (thinly sliced)
- ¼ cup Sliced Almonds
- ¼ cup Parmesan (grated)
- 2 cloves Garlic (sliced)
- 2 Tbsps. Olive Oil
- 1 tsp Crushed Red Pepper Flakes
- Salt & Pepper to taste

Method

1. In a large bowl, toss squash with 1 teaspoon salt. Let stand 10 minutes. Squeeze squash to remove moisture. Toast almonds in a dry pan on medium heat for 3 minutes. Toss occasionally. Set aside. Heat oil in the same pan over medium heat. Add pepper flakes and garlic. Cook 2 minutes.

2. Add squash. Cook 5 minutes, tossing occasionally. Gradually add in parmesan. Season with salt and pepper. Gradually add in almonds. Serve.

3 Ways to Spice Up This Dish

Add chopped jalapeno and lime juice in place of almonds and cheese. Add grated carrot, rice vinegar, and miso instead of cheese. Add cumin and coriander. Dollop with Greek yogurt before serving.

173. Berry Pudding

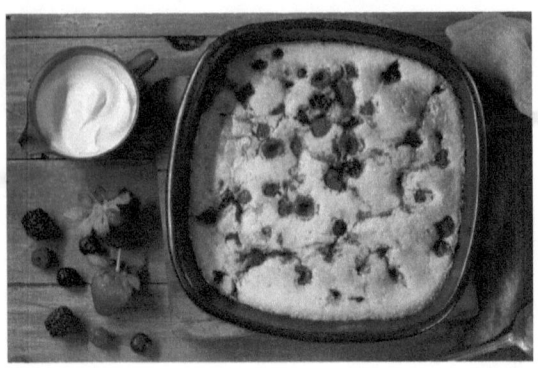

Summary

Celebrate the berry season with this simple pudding.

Ingredients

- 1 (1 lbs.) loaf Brioche or Challah Bread (cut into 1" slices)
- 2 pints Strawberries (quartered)
- 2 pints Blueberries
- 2 pints Blackberries
- 2 pints Raspberries
- 1 cup Sugar
- 1 Vanilla Bean (split lengthwise)
- 6 Tbsps. Butter
- ½ tsp Cinnamon

Method

1. Line a pan with plastic wrap. Place pan on a baking sheet. In a pot, mix together all berries, ½ cup water, and 1 cup sugar. Simmer 10 minutes, stirring often. Set aside. Spread butter onto bread slices. Mix 2 tablespoons sugar with cinnamon. Sprinkle over buttered bread. Drizzle ½ cup berry sauce in bottom of lined pan.

2. Arrange a single layer of bread slices in pan. Pour 1 ½ cups berry sauce over bread. Repeat this layering until ingredients are used up. Cover with plastic. Set a plate in the pan and weigh it down with heavy cans. Chill 1 hour.

Health Benefits of Berries

Improves brain health and cognitive function. Help control appetite and manage weight. Helps prevent age-related illnesses like Alzheimer's.

174. Corn & Cod Chowder

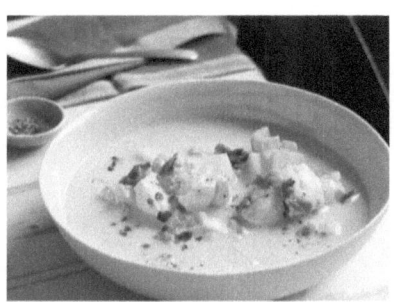

Summary

Lighten up a heavy chowder with corn and cod.

Ingredients

- 3 slices Bacon (Halved)
- 8 Scallions (sliced)
- ¾ lbs. Cod (skin removed, chopped)
- 2 ½ cups Corn Kernels
- ¼ cup Half and Half
- 2 Potatoes (peeled, diced)
- 2 cups Whole Milk
- 2 cups Chicken Broth
- 1 ½ tsp Garlic (chopped)
- 2 Tbsps. Flour
- 2 tsp Thyme
- Salt & Pepper to taste

Method

1. In a large pan, cook bacon on medium heat for 6 minutes. Let bacon drain on paper towels. Cook scallions in bacon grease 2 minutes. Add garlic. Cook 1 minute.

2. Add flour. Cook 2 minutes, stirring constantly. Stir in milk, broth, potatoes, thyme, salt and pepper. Bring to a boil. Reduce heat to medium-low. Simmer 10 minutes. Stir in cod, corn, and 2 slices of bacon. Simmer 5 minutes. Stir in half and half. Simmer 2 minutes. Crumble remaining slice of bacon. Ladle chowder into bowls. Garnish with bacon crumbles.

Health Benefits of Cod

A great low-cholesterol source of protein. High in B vitamins (including the essential B12). High in cholesterol-lowering niacin.

175. Fruit Cobbler

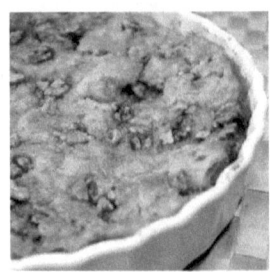

Summary

Treat yourself to a summery cobbler with nectarines and raspberries.

Ingredients

- 4 cups Nectarines (peeled, sliced)
- 1-pint Raspberries
- 2/3 cup Sugar
- 1 ¼ cup Flour
- ½ cup Cornmeal
- 6 Tbsps. Buttermilk
- 5 Tbsps. Butter (sliced)
- 2 Tbsps. Cornstarch
- 1 Tbsp. Raw Sugar
- 1 Tbsp. Fresh Lemon Juice
- 2 tsp Baking Powder
- ¾ tsp Salt
- ½ tsp Baking Soda

Method

1. Preheat oven to 375°F. In a bowl, toss together raspberries, nectarines, cornstarch, juice, ¼ teaspoon salt, and 1/3 cup sugar. Add mixture to a greased baking dish. In another bowl, whisk together remaining sugar, cornmeal, baking powder, baking soda, flour, and ½ teaspoon salt. Add flour mixture to food processor with butter. Pulse until dough forms pea-sized pieces.

2. Add buttermilk. Pulse until combined. Measure out 1/3 cup portions of dough to create 10 round biscuits. Place biscuits on top of fruit mixture in baking dish. Lightly press biscuits down with fingers. Sprinkle the top with raw sugar. Bake 50 minutes.

Health Benefits of Nectarines

High in antioxidants. Helps maintain collagen and prevent wrinkles. Improves digestion and helps weight loss.

176. Summer Stir Fry

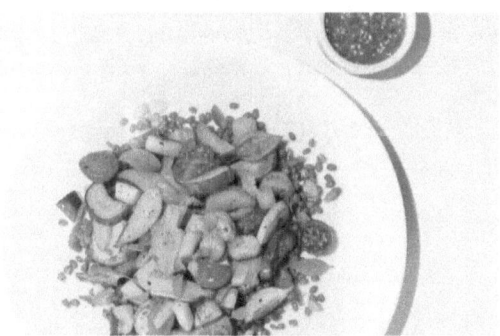

Summary

This lively dish is full of bold and vibrant flavors.

Ingredients

- 4 cups Mixed Summer Veggies (chopped)
- 3 cups Mixed Fresh Herbs (your preference)
- 2 cups Quinoa (cooked)
- ½ cup Scallions (sliced)
- 1 ½" piece Ginger (peeled, sliced)
- 1 clove Garlic

- 7 Tbsps. Olive Oil
- 2 Tbsps. Rice Vinegar
- 2 Tbsps. Sesame Seeds
- Salt & Pepper to taste

Method

1. Pulse together garlic, ginger, ¼ cup scallions, and 2 cups herbs in a processor. Add 4 tablespoons oil, ¼ cup water, and vinegar. Pulse until pureed. Transfer to a bowl and stir in sesame seeds. Season with salt and pepper. Heat 1 tablespoon oil in a large pan on medium-high heat. Add remaining scallions and quinoa. Stir fry 3 minutes. Season with salt and pepper. Divide quinoa mix into serving bowls.

2. Return skillet to heat. Add 2 tablespoons oil. Add all vegetables. Season with salt and pepper. Stir fry 4 minutes. Add 1 cup fresh herbs. Toss to combine. Divide vegetable mix into bowls with quinoa. Drizzle herb sauce over the top.

More Health Benefits of Herbs

Fresh oregano is a natural anti-inflammatory. Fresh thyme is high in vitamins A & C as well as iron. Fresh sage is the herb with the most antioxidants.

177. Summery Linguine

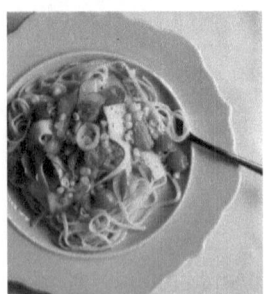

Summary

This linguine gets a summer makeover with corn, tomato, and fresh basil.

Ingredients

- 8 oz. Linguine
- 2 ½ cups Corn Kernels

- 1 ¾ cups Sugar Snap Peas (string-less)
- ½ lbs. Small Tomatoes
- 1 ¼ cup Fresh Basil (chopped)
- ¾ cup Parmesan (grated)
- 3 Tbsps. Olive Oil

Method

1. Boil linguine until al dente. Drain. Reserve 1 cup of liquid. Place ½ cup liquid in blender. Add ½ cup corn. Blend until smooth. Heat oil in large pan on medium heat. Add peas and 2 cups corn. Sprinkle in salt and pepper. Cover and cook 5 minutes, stirring often. Add pasta, corn puree, tomatoes, parmesan, and basil. Toss until pasta is thoroughly coated.

Health Benefits of Snap Peas

High in vitamin K. High in B vitamins. High in folate.

178. Summer Tarts

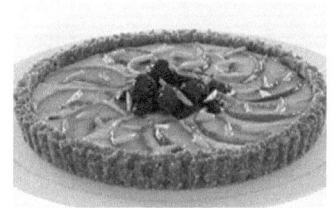

Summary

These savory tarts are a great appetizer for a summer barbecue.

Ingredients

- 2 ½ cups Whole Grain Flour
- 2 sticks Cold Butter (diced)
- 5-8 Tbsps. Water
- ½ tsp Salt
- ¾ cup Whole Milk
- ¾ cup Heavy Cream
- 3 large Eggs
- 1 large Egg Yolk
- 12 Green Beans (trimmed, chopped)

- 12 Grape Tomatoes (halved)
- 6 (¼") slices Goat Cheese
- 2 tsp Chives (chopped)

Method

1. Blend together butter, salt, and flour in a bowl. Mix with fingers until roughly mixed. Drizzle in 5 tablespoons cold water. Stir with a fork until mixed. If dough doesn't hold together when squeezed, add more cold water ½ tablespoon at a time. Turn dough onto floured surface. Divide into 4 pieces.

2. Press dough out to help distribute butter fat. Gather dough together and form into 2 (5") squares. Wrap in plastic wrap. Chill 1 hour. Arrange 6 flan rings on a baking sheet lined with parchment paper. Roll out chilled dough on a floured surface until it is a 10"x16" rectangle. Cut into 6 squares. Gently fit each pastry square into each flan ring. Trim excess dough so that it is flush with the rim. Gently prick the pastry shells with a fork. Chill 30 minutes. Preheat oven to 375°F. Line shells with foil and place weights in each ring. Bake 20 minutes.

3. Remove weights and foil. Let cool. Reduce oven to 350°F. Boil green beans 3 minutes. Drain and spoon into tart shells. Spoon in tomatoes. Top with round of goat cheese. Whisk together milk, cream, eggs, and egg yolks. Sprinkle in salt and pepper. Divide evenly among tarts. Bake 20 minutes or until custard sets.

Health Benefits of Whole Grains

High in both protein and fiber, helping to control appetite and speed up weight loss. Specifically helps reduce belly fat. Help stabilize blood sugar levels.

179. Summer Garden Tortellini

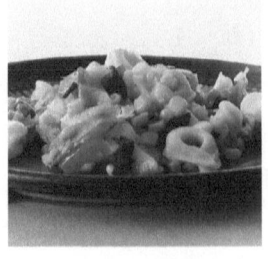

Summary

Brighten up your tortellini with the taste of summer.

Ingredients

- 8 oz. Dried Cheese Tortellini
- 2 cups Corn Kernels
- 2 Tomatoes (chopped)
- 2 oz. Prosciutto Slices (cut into strips)
- 1 clove Garlic (chopped)
- ½ cup Fresh Basil (chopped)
- ½ stick Butter

Method

1. Cook tortellini in boiling water. In a pan on medium-high heat, cook prosciutto, garlic, butter, salt and pepper 5 minutes. In a large bowl, combine tomatoes with corn mixture. Drain tortellini. Reserve ¼ cup pasta water. Mix tortellini, basil and ¼ cup water in with vegetables. Mix well. Season with salt and pepper.

Health Benefits of Basil

Acts as a natural antibacterial. High in vitamin K. High in magnesium and manganese.

180. Summer Kebabs

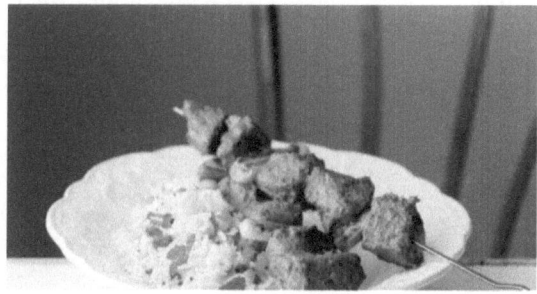

Summary

These chicken and summer veggie kebabs come with a fresh salad on the side for a complete summer meal.

Ingredients

- 5 cups Arugula
- 2 cups Cherry Tomatoes (halved)
- 1 ½ lbs. Boneless Skinless Chicken Breasts (cubed)
- ½ cup Olive Oil
- ¼ cup Balsamic Vinegar
- 1 Red Onion (cut into wedges)
- 2 large Zucchini (cubed)
- 2 Yellow Squash (cubed)
- 1 Orange (juice, zest)
- 1 Lemon (juice, zest)
- 1 Lime (juice, zest)
- 2 tsp Cumin
- 2 tsp Chili Powder
- Pepper to taste

Method

1. Soak wooden skewers in water 20 minutes. Whisk together ¼ cup oil with the juice and zest from orange, lemon, and lime. Whisk in the cumin and chili powder. Add chicken. Stir to coat. Cover with plastic wrap. Marinate 1 hour.

2. Whisk together ¼ cup oil with vinegar. Coat vegetables with oil-vinegar mixture. Stick the chicken and vegetables onto the skewers in an alternating pattern. Season with pepper. Heat grill to medium-high heat. Cook kebabs about 7 minutes per side (or until chicken is cooked through). Toss arugula with remaining oil-vinegar mixture. Salt and pepper to taste.

Health Benefits of Olive Oil

High in unsaturated fats which help you absorb nutrients and stay full for longer. Improves circulation. Can act as a natural pain reliever.

181. Squash Sloppy Joes

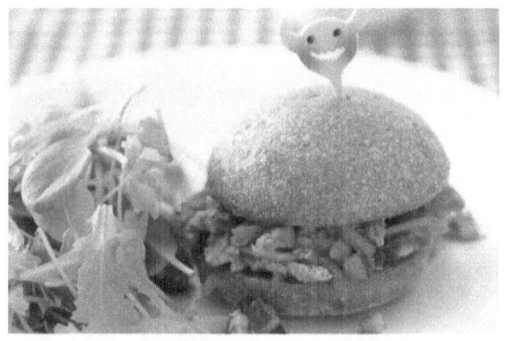

Summary

Add new flavors (and more nutritional value) to sloppy joes with this recipe.

Ingredients

- 6 Hamburger Buns
- 1 lbs. Ground Beef
- 1 ½ cups Summer Squash (diced)
- 1 carrot (chopped)
- ½ Onion (chopped)
- 1 (6oz.) can Tomato Paste
- 3 cloves Garlic (minced)
- 3 oz. Cheddar (sliced)
- 1 Tbsp. Chili Powder
- 1 tsp Paprika
- 1 tsp Oregano
- Salt & Pepper to taste

Method

1. Preheat broiler. Brown beef in a pan over medium-high heat. Add onion. Cook 2 minutes. Add carrot. Cook 2 minutes. Add squash. Cook 1 minute. Stir in tomato paste and 1 ½ cups water. Stir until dissolved.

2. Add garlic, paprika, chili powder, oregano, salt, and pepper. Reduce heat to medium. Cook 8-10 minutes. Place cheese slices on bottom halves of buns. Toast both sides of buns in broiler (until cheese is melted). Remove buns. Fill sandwiches with meat mixture.

Health Benefits of Summer Squash

Lots of lutein and zeaxanthin for eye health. High in tumor-fighting nasunin. High in red blood cell producing B vitamins.

182. Drunken Shaved Ice

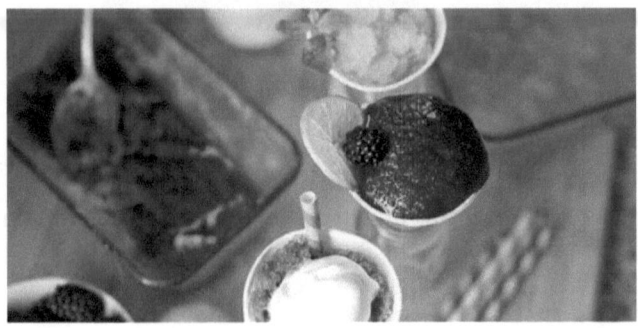

Summary

There's no better way to cool off than with spiked shaved ice!

Ingredients

- 4 cups Shaved Ice
- 1 cup Campari (chilled)

Method

1. Pack 1 cup shaved ice into each cocktail glass. Drizzle with chilled Campari.

Try Replacing Campari with

A combination of dark rum, apple cider, and lemon juice. Tequila and your favorite margarita mix. A blend of peach nectar, bourbon, mint simple syrup, and lemon juice.

183. Mint Hot Fudge Sundaes

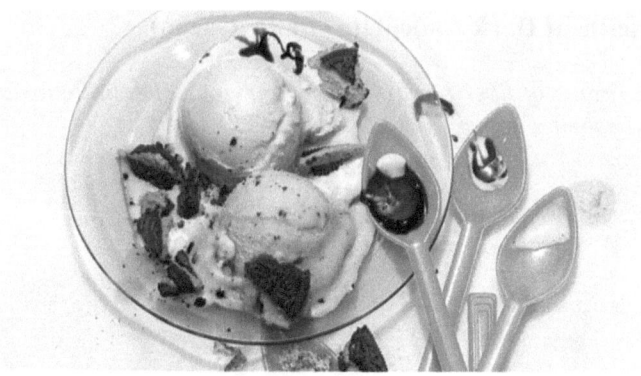

Summary

This sundae is soothing and refreshing all at the same time.

Ingredients

- 1-pint Vanilla Ice Cream
- 1-pint Mint Ice Cream
- 10 Mint Chocolate Oreos (broken)
- 1 cup Dark Chocolate Chunks
- ¼ cup Sugar
- ¼ cup Water
- 1 oz. Unsweetened Chocolate (chopped)
- 2 Tbsps. Fresh Mint
- 1 Tbsp. Sugar
- 2 Tbsps. Butter
- ½ tsp Peppermint Extract
- Sweetened Whipped Cream

Method

1. In a small pan over medium-high heat, stir together ¼ cup sugar with butter, water, and dark chocolate chunks. Stir in unsweetened chocolate and peppermint extract until smooth. Set aside.

2. In a bowl, toss together mint and 1 tablespoon sugar. Set aside. Place a scoop of vanilla in each bowl. Top with broken cookies. Scoop in mint ice cream. Top with more cookies. Drizzle the chocolate sauce over. Top with whipped cream. Garnish with mint sugar.

Health Benefits of Dark Chocolate (70%+ Cacao)

Contains 11 grams of fiber per 100 grams serving. Rich in antioxidants. High in iron, magnesium, copper, and manganese.

184. Whiskey Wings

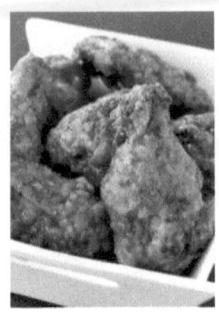

Summary

Whiskey adds a new dimension to these scrumptious wings.

Ingredients

- 24 Chicken Wings
- ¼ cup Dijon Mustard
- ¾ cup BBQ Sauce
- ¼ cup Whiskey
- 1 Tbsp. Sugar
- Salt & Pepper to taste

Method

1. Cut each wing in half and remove the drumettes. Discard drumettes. Rinse wings well. Pat dry. Season with salt and pepper. Set aside in a Ziploc bag.

2. In a small pan, whisk together sugar and whiskey. Simmer on medium-high heat. Remove from heat. Whisk in mustard. Cool. Pour the mixture into the bag with the wings. Seal the bag. Toss to coat. Let marinate 30 minutes in the freezer. Prepare the grill for smoking at medium-low heat. Place wings in a shallow aluminum pan. Place pan in grill. Cook 2 hours.

Health Benefits of Whiskey

Contains heart-healthy antioxidants. May help prevent Alzheimer's and dementia. Helps lower stress.

*high quality whiskeys in moderation.

185. Fruit Salad in Herbed Syrup

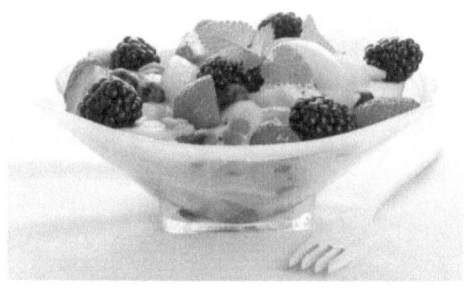

Summary

This unique variation on fruit salad is light and refreshing.

Ingredients

- 1-pint Strawberries (halved)
- ½ pint Raspberries
- ½ pint Blueberries
- 2 Oranges (peeled, sectioned)
- 2 Kiwis (peeled, sliced)
- 1 Mango (peeled, pitted, cubed)
- 1 Papaya (peeled, pitted, cubed)
- 2 cups Pineapple Chunks
- 1 cup Cantaloupe (cubed)
- 1 cup Sugar
- 1 cup Water
- ¼ cup Fresh Rosemary
- ¼ cup Fresh Mint (julienned)
- 1 sprig Rosemary
- 1 sprig Mint

Method

1. In a small pot, combine 1 cup water, 1 cup sugar, ¼ cup rosemary, and ¼ cup mint. Bring to a boil. Stir until sugar is dissolved. Remove herbs. Set aside. Combine all the fruits into a large bowl. Pour herbed syrup mixture over and mix well. Garnish with rosemary and mint sprigs.

Health Benefits of Pineapple

Improves immune system. High in bone-strengthening manganese. Improves gum health.

186. Blueberry Banana Bread

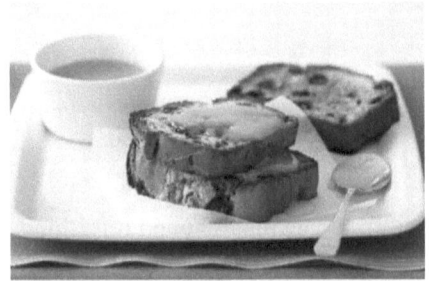

Summary

This simple quick bread makes an excellent addition to a relaxing Sunday brunch.

Ingredients

- ¾ cup Buttermilk
- ¾ cup Brown Sugar
- ¼ cup Olive Oil
- 1 cup Bananas (mashed)
- 2 ¼ cups Whole Grain Flour
- 1 ¼ cup Blueberries
- 2 large Eggs
- ¾ tsp Cinnamon
- 1 ½ tsp Baking Soda
- ¼ tsp Nutmeg
- ½ tsp Salt

Method

1. Preheat oven to 375°F. Whisk together buttermilk, brown sugar, eggs, and oil. Stir in bananas. In another bowl, whisk together flour, baking soda, cinnamon, baking soda, nutmeg, and salt.

2. Stir the dry ingredients into the wet ingredients until combined. Add blueberries. Pour mixture into a greased baking dish. Bake until golden brown and cooked through (about 50 minutes). Cool 10 minutes.

Health Benefits of Bananas

Helps treat symptoms of depression. Eaten before workouts, helps prevent muscle cramps. Boost immune system.

187. Frozen Peach Yogurt

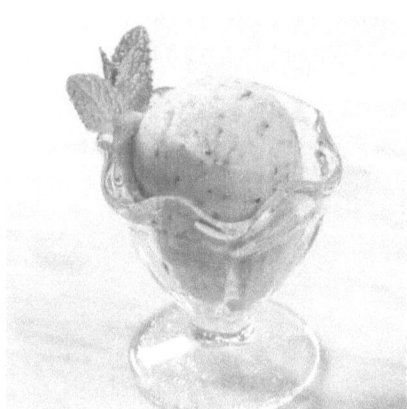

Summary

This simple alternative is a great alternative to ice cream on a hot day.

Ingredients

- 3 ½ cups Frozen Peaches (chopped)
- ½ cup Sugar
- ½ cup Plain Greek Yogurt
- 1 Tbsp. Fresh Lemon Juice

Method

1. In a food processor, pulse together peaches and sugars. In a bowl, combine yogurt and lemon juice. Pour the yogurt into the processor in batches. Process until smooth and creamy.

Health Benefits of Peaches

Helps maintain collagen and moisture in the skin. Helps slow down hair loss and rejuvenate scalp. Helps lower anxiety.

Final Words

I would like to thank you for downloading my book and I hope I have been able to help you and educate you about something new.

If you have enjoyed this book and would like to share your positive thoughts, could you please take 30 seconds of your time to go back and give me a review on my Amazon book page!

I greatly appreciate seeing these reviews because it helps me share my hard work!

Again, thank you and I wish you all the best with your cooking journey!

Last Chance to Get YOUR Bonus!

FOR A LIMITED TIME ONLY – Get Olivia's best-selling book *"The #1 Cookbook: Over 170+ of the Most Popular Recipes Across 7 Different Cuisines!"* absolutely FREE!

Readers have absolutely loved this book because of the wide variety of recipes. It is highly recommended you check these recipes out and see what you can add to your home menu!

Once again, as a big thank-you for downloading this book, I'd like to offer it to you *100% FREE for a LIMITED TIME ONLY!*

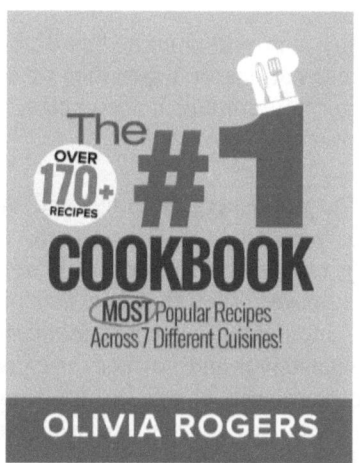

Get your free copy at:

TheMenuAtHome.com/Bonus

Disclaimer

This book and related site provides recipe and food advice in an informative and educational manner only, with information that is general in nature and that is not specific to you, the reader. The contents of this book and related site are intended to assist you and other readers in your personal efforts. Consult your physician or nutritionist regarding the applicability of any information provided in our information to you.

Nothing in this book should be construed as personal advice or diagnosis, and must not be used in this manner. The information provided about conditions is general in nature. This information does not cover all possible uses, actions, precautions, side-effects, or interactions of medicines, or medical procedures. The information in this site should not be considered as complete and does not cover all diseases, ailments, physical conditions, or their treatment.

No Warranties: The authors and publishers don't guarantee or warrant the quality, accuracy, completeness, timeliness, appropriateness or suitability of the information in this book, or of any product or services referenced by this site.

The information in this site is provided on an "as is" basis and the authors and publishers make no representations or warranties of any kind with respect to this information. This site may contain inaccuracies, typographical errors, or other errors.

Liability Disclaimer: The publishers, authors, and other parties involved in the creation, production, provision of information, or delivery of this site specifically disclaim any responsibility, and shall not be held liable for any damages, claims, injuries, losses, liabilities, costs, or obligations including any direct, indirect, special, incidental, or consequences damages (collectively known as "Damages") whatsoever and howsoever caused, arising out of, or in connection with the use or misuse of the site and the information contained within it, whether such Damages arise in contract, tort, negligence, equity, statute law, or by way of other legal theory.